Mathematics for Nurses

Second Edition

Mathematics for Nurses

Second Edition

Grace G. Johnson, R.N., B.S., M.S.N.
Associate Professor of Nursing
Houston Baptist University
Houston, Texas

A̅C̲C̲ APPLETON-CENTURY-CROFTS / Norwalk, Connecticut

Copyright © 1986 by Appleton-Century-Crofts
A Publishing Division of Prentice-Hall, Inc.

86 87 88 89 90 / 10 9 8 7 6 5 4 3 2 1

Prentice-Hall of Australia, Pty. Ltd., Sydney
Prentice-Hall Canada, Inc.
Prentice-Hall Hispanoamericana, S.A., Mexico
Prentice-Hall of India Private Limited, New Delhi
Prentice-Hall International (UK) Limited, London
Prentice-Hall of Japan, Inc., Tokyo
Prentice-Hall of Southeast Asia (Pte.) Ltd., Singapore
Whitehall Books Ltd., Wellington, New Zealand
Editora Prentice-Hall do Brasil Ltda., Rio de Janeiro

Library of Congress Cataloging-in-Publication Data

Johnson, Grace G.
    Mathematics for nurses.

    Includes index.
      1. Pharmaceutical arithmetic—Programmed instruction.
2. Nursing—Mathematics—Programmed instruction.
I. Title. [DNLM: 1. Drugs—administration & dosage—
nurses' instruction. 2. Drugs—administration & dosage—
programmed instruction. 3. Mathematics—nurses' instruction. 4 Mathematics—programmed instruction.
QV 18 J67m]
RS57.J64 1985   615.5'8   85-15746
ISBN 0-8385-6175-6

Design: M. Chandler Martylewski

PRINTED IN THE UNITED STATES OF AMERICA

CONTENTS

v

PREFACE

This book is designed as a self-instructional unit which may be learned at the individual's own rate of speed, or it may be used as a regular text in a classroom setting. It is written primarily for students in professional nursing programs but may be used equally well in licensed vocational nursing programs, for inservice education programs and refresher courses, or as a desk reference for nurses who administer medications on hospital units, in clinics or offices, or wherever they are employed.

Formulas have been limited and simplified as much as possible to make calculations easier. Examples of problems for each formula are worked to show the student all possibilities for use of the formula.

Practice problems and additional practice problems follow each lesson. Solving the problems is a part of the learning experience, and it is strongly recommended that the student work and *understand* the problems assigned. It is most important that one learn the material and understand the mathematics involved so that medications can be administered quickly and correctly. Some practice problems are more difficult than those usually encountered. They are included to improve problem-solving ability. They are not the usual problems that one will be solving every day.

It is recommended that practice problems and tests be worked at the proficiency level and conditions given; however, instructors may set their own limits and proficiency level.

The first lesson focuses on review of arithmetic. After mastering these mathematical skills the student is then prepared to practice his or her computation skills by converting from one system to another, and then by calculating actual dosage and solution problems.

Review lessons are included to reinforce learning. Lessons 15 through 20 are placed in the back of the book as this content is rarely practiced by nurses today. They are included for reference, and practice problems are included to prepare the student for those rare instances when a nurse might have to compute dosages for injections using tablets, measure minims, or prepare solutions from pure drugs.

Although the Metric system has been adopted almost universally, some physicians still write orders in the Apothecaries' system; therefore, the Apothecaries' tables and practice problems for the Apothecaries' system are included.

Calculators may not be used to solve problems because they will not always be readily available for everyone, and because the student would not become proficient in solving problems.

Each lesson is preceded by objectives that let the student know exactly what is to be learned. The lessons are designed to be completed sequentially. For example, the objectives for Lesson 1 should be achieved before proceeding to Lesson 2; Lesson 2 objectives should be completed before going to Lesson 3, etc.

There are 78 problems in the Pretest. If you miss no more than 8, you may omit Lesson 1, Review of Arithmetic, and proceed to Lesson 2. However, you may find the review helpful later.

Since only basic, pertinent information is presented in these lessons, please contact the instructor at any time for additional help, or clarification of problems or information.

INTRODUCTION

One important responsibility of the nurse is the administration of medications and the preparation of certain solutions of different strengths for use in various treatments. In order to prepare these medications and solutions, the nurse must be able to do a few mathematical calculations using the simple arithmetic that was studied in grade school. This includes addition, subtraction, multiplication, and division since these concepts are used in dealing with fractions, decimals, percentage, ratio, and proportion.

Since this material is presented in small steps in the simplest manner possible, and students are informed immediately of the correctness of their answers, learning will be both enhanced and reinforced. Because of the diversity of backgrounds in mathematics among nursing students, independent participation and advancement should be promoted through self-instructional methods.

Most of us do not appreciate the need for learning certain things when the opportunity arises, and instead learn only for today's lesson or tomorrow's test. Since a knowledge of mathematical calculations is needed throughout one's nursing career, as well as in life generally, the student should come to class with the idea that he or she does want to learn and can master the simple arithmetic required for computing dosage and preparing solutions.

Difficulty with arithmetic is frequently due to some form of carelessness; e.g., failure to add or subtract correctly, failure to read carefully, or failure to transpose the problem correctly. Mistakes in administering medications and computing dosage may be dangerous, for we are not dealing with money, apples, pies, but instead, with human lives. If the patient's safety and comfort are not endangered through error, certainly the physician's plan for treating the patient may be altered and the rate of recovery may be delayed.

If a patient is given an incorrect dosage or the wrong medication, it matters little as to the cause—misreading, carelessness in arithmetic—any mistake involves risk to that patient. Any problem that you solve, even though it is only on paper, is wrong unless it is correct in every detail.

If you begin now by following the simple rules listed below, you will find that when you are ready to prepare medications you will have much less difficulty in solving problems and very few inaccuracies.

1. *Read accurately and carefully.* Check the name and dosage of medication at least three times before solving your problems. For example, if you read "morphine 0.016 g" as "morphine 0.16 g" and calculate accordingly, you are giving the patient ten times the amount of drug he should receive, which would be a fatal dose.

2. *Always assume your answer to be incorrect and recheck several times.* Ask yourself these questions: "Is my answer logical?" "Does it make sense?" For example, suppose you are asked to solve for x in $1/2x = 50$. Logic tells you that if $1/2x = 50$, x must be greater than 50. Therefore, if your answer is 50 or less, you know that it is incorrect.

3. *Think clearly.* You must not only read carefully and accurately, and follow what you have read exactly, but you must concentrate on each step of your problem. When you are preparing medications, focus your mind only on what you are doing. *Do not talk to anyone, and do not let anyone talk to you.*

4. *Reread statement of problem and ask yourself if you have done what is asked of you.* If you are preparing an injection, for example, your answer will be in minims or milliliters and not grains or grams.

5. *Learn formulas and tables.* Problem solving will be simple if you master the formulas and tables as they are given.

6. *Solve your problems the "easy" way.* Study the problem carefully and solve it by the simplest method for *you.*

7. *Draw pictures to clarify the problem.* For example, if you are having trouble solving a problem involving fractions $(1/8 + 3/8)$, try drawing a pie that is divided into the appropriate number of parts. In this case, the pie would have eight parts and you would quickly see that four parts equal 1/2 of the pie.

PRETEST

The following pretest is designed to assess the student's basic knowledge of arithmetic and to determine whether the review in Lesson 1 is necessary.

Write as Roman numerals:

1. 9 _____   2. 29 _____   3. 44 _____

Write as Arabic numbers:

4. XLVIII _____   5. XXXIX _____   6. XLIX _____

Multiply:

7. 1.004×0.02 _____   8. 3000×0.04 _____

9. 5302×0.12 _____

Divide:

10. 636.24 by 0.12 _____   11. 30.15 by 0.15 _____

12. 0.004 by 0.2 _____

Arrange in order, largest value first:

13. $\dfrac{1}{10}, \dfrac{3}{20}, \dfrac{4}{5}, \dfrac{3}{4}, \dfrac{1}{2}$

14. $\dfrac{1}{100}, \dfrac{1}{150}, \dfrac{1}{75}, \dfrac{1}{130}, \dfrac{1}{200}$

15. $\dfrac{1}{6}, \dfrac{2}{3}, \dfrac{3}{4}, \dfrac{5}{8}, \dfrac{5}{6}$

Multiply:

16. $\dfrac{1}{100} \times \dfrac{1}{2} \times 50$ _____   17. $2 \times \dfrac{1}{4} \times \dfrac{1}{3}$ _____

18. $\dfrac{1}{20} \times \dfrac{1}{3} \times 60$ _____

Divide:

19. $2\frac{1}{3}$ by $\dfrac{1}{6}$ _____   20. $\dfrac{1}{100}$ by 5 _____

21. $12\frac{1}{4}$ by $3\frac{1}{2}$ _____

Add:

22. $\dfrac{1}{6} + \dfrac{1}{8} + \dfrac{2}{3} + \dfrac{3}{16}$ _____

23. $\dfrac{1}{4} + \dfrac{3}{12} + \dfrac{5}{6} + \dfrac{1}{8}$ _____

24. $\dfrac{3}{4} + \dfrac{3}{16} + \dfrac{5}{8} + \dfrac{3}{32}$ _____

Subtract:

25. $\dfrac{8}{15} - \dfrac{1}{3}$ _____   26. $\dfrac{1}{16} - \dfrac{1}{64}$ _____

27. $\dfrac{3}{4} - \dfrac{1}{6}$ _____

Change to common fractions:

28. 0.2 _____   29. 0.008 _____   30. 0.05 _____

Change to decimal fractions:

31. $\dfrac{3}{4}$ _____   32. $\dfrac{1}{4}$ _____

33. $\dfrac{1}{200}$ _____

Change to decimal fractions:

34. 5% _____   35. 50% _____   36. $\frac{1}{2}\%$ _____

Change to percents:

37. $\dfrac{1}{4}$ _____   38. $\dfrac{1}{20}$ _____   39. $\dfrac{1}{2}$ _____

Express as ratios:

40. $\dfrac{1}{100}$ _____   41. $\dfrac{1}{20}$ _____   42. $\dfrac{1}{50}$ _____

Circle the larger fraction:

43. $\dfrac{1}{4}$ or $\dfrac{1}{6}$ 44. $\dfrac{3}{8}$ or $\dfrac{3}{4}$

45. $\dfrac{1}{60}$ or $\dfrac{1}{25}$ 46. $\dfrac{1}{100}$ or $\dfrac{1}{150}$

Find the value of x:

47. $x : 1000 :: \dfrac{1}{2} : 100$ 50. $\dfrac{1}{4} : 100 :: \dfrac{1}{10} : x$

48. $5 : 1000 :: x : 100$ 51. $x : 50 :: \dfrac{1}{4} : \dfrac{1}{2}$

49. $x : 1000 :: \dfrac{1}{100} : \dfrac{1}{1000}$ 52. $x : 0.05 :: 10 : 100$

Express the given numbers in alternate form:

Fraction	Decimal Fraction	Percent	Ratio
53. $\dfrac{1}{1000}$	54. _____	55. _____	56. _____
57. _____	58. 0.5	59. _____	60. _____
61. _____	62. _____	63. $\frac{1}{2}\%$	64. _____
65. _____	66. _____	67. _____	68. 1 : 25
69. _____	70. _____	71. 5%	72. _____

73. A 1% solution contains how many parts of drug in every 100 equal parts of water? _____ .

74. A tablet has grain $\frac{1}{100}$ of drug. How much of the drug is contained in one-half of the tablet? _____

75. An ounce of solution contains 32 grains of drug. What fraction of an ounce would contain 8 grains? _____

76. One tablet has grain $\frac{1}{6}$ of drug. How many grains are contained in two tablets? _____

77. How many sixths equal $\frac{1}{2}$? _____

78. Which is larger: 0.01 or 0.016? _____

Answers to Pretest

1. IX	2. XXIX	3. XLIV
4. 48	5. 39	6. 49
7. 0.02008	8. 120	9. 636.24
10. 5302	11. 201	12. 0.02

13. $\frac{4}{5}, \frac{3}{4}, \frac{1}{2}, \frac{3}{20}, \frac{1}{10}$ 14. $\frac{1}{75}, \frac{1}{100}, \frac{1}{130}, \frac{1}{150}, \frac{1}{200}$

15. $\frac{5}{6}, \frac{3}{4}, \frac{2}{3}, \frac{5}{8}, \frac{1}{6}$

16. $\frac{1}{4}$ 17. $\frac{1}{6}$ 18. 1

19. 14   20. $\frac{1}{500}$ 21. $3\frac{1}{2}$

22. $1\frac{7}{48}$ 23. $1\frac{11}{24}$ 24. $1\frac{21}{32}$

25. $\frac{3}{15}$ or $\frac{1}{5}$ 26. $\frac{3}{64}$ 27. $\frac{7}{12}$

28. $\frac{2}{10}$ or $\frac{1}{5}$ 29. $\frac{8}{1000}$ or $\frac{1}{125}$ 30. $\frac{5}{100}$ or $\frac{1}{20}$

31. 0.75	32. 0.25	33. 0.005
34. 0.05	35. 0.5	36. 0.005
37. 25%	38. 5%	39. 50%
40. 1 : 100	41. 1 : 20	42. 1 : 50

43. $\dfrac{1}{4}$ 44. $\dfrac{3}{4}$ 45. $\dfrac{1}{25}$

46. $\dfrac{1}{100}$ 47. 5   48. 0.5

49. 10,000   50. 40   51. 25

52. 0.005

53. $\dfrac{1}{1000}$ 54. 0.001   55. 0.1%   56. 1 : 1000

57. $\dfrac{1}{2}$ 58. 0.5   59. 50%   60. 1 : 2

61. $\dfrac{1}{200}$ 62. 0.005   63. $\frac{1}{2}$%   64. 1 : 200

65. $\dfrac{1}{25}$ 66. 0.04   67. 4%   68. 1 : 25

69. $\dfrac{1}{20}$ 70. 0.05   71. 5%   72. 1 : 20

73. 1 part   74. $\dfrac{1}{200}$

75. $\dfrac{1}{4}$ ounce   76. grain $\dfrac{1}{3}$

77. 3   78. 0.016

If you made no more than eight errors, you may omit Lesson 1 and go on to Lesson 2. However, you may find the review in Lesson 1 helpful later.

LESSON 1

Review of Arithmetic

Objectives

After completing this lesson, the student will be able to:

- Recall concepts of basic arithmetic to solve problems using fractions, decimal fractions, percentage, ratio, and proportion.

- Apply these concepts to the preparation of medications and solutions.

- Arrange a set of decimal fractions in order of magnitude.

- Arrange a set of fractions in order of magnitude.

- State seven rules that will help in solving problems and in preventing errors.

- State rules for changing from one number form to another:
  a. Percent to decimal fraction, fraction, and ratio.
  b. Decimal fraction to percent, fraction, and ratio.
  c. Fraction to decimal fraction, percent, and ratio.
  d. Ratio to fraction, decimal fraction, and percent.

- Demonstrate an understanding of basic arithmetic by solving the practice problems at the end of this lesson with no more than nine errors.

ROMAN NUMERALS

Roman numerals from 1 to 100 are used as units of the Apothecaries' system of weights and measures; therefore, the nurse must know how to write or read all numbers from 1 to 100 as Roman numerals. The basic Roman numerals are expressed by seven capital letters:

1—I	10—X	100—C	1000—M
5—V	50—L	500—D	

Lower case rather than capital Roman numerals are used to express dosage in the Apothecaries' system; eg, *iv* rather than *IV.* As a check, the Roman numeral *i* is always written with a dot over it when lower-case numbers are used (*iii*). The shorter form should be used in writing a numeral. Thus, *xvvi* is incorrect and should be written *xxi*; similarly, *xiiii* is incorrect and should be written *xiv*.

Expressing Roman Numerals

In writing Roman numerals there are several rules to follow:

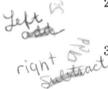

1. Numerals are never repeated more than three times in a sequence.
   Example: III = 3, XXX = 30, while 40 is expressed as XL
2. When a symbol of less value follows, or is to the right of a larger value, you add the values.
   Example: VII = 5 + 1 + 1 = 7
3. When a symbol of less value precedes, or is to the left of a larger value, you subtract the values.
   Example: IX = 10 − 1 = 9, or XLI = 50 − 10 + 1 = 41
4. When a smaller numeral is between two numerals of greater value, the smaller numeral is subtracted from the numeral following it.
   Example: XIX = 10 + (10 − 1) = 19 or, MCMXLVI = First M = 1000; then subtract 100 (C) from the second 1000 (M) = 900; then subtract 10 (X) from 50 (L) = 40 and add V and I = 6; then add all together: 1000 + 900 + 40 + 6 = 1946.

PROBLEM 1*: Write the following as Roman numerals:

a. 14	b. 44	c. 49
d. 62	e. 83	f. 99

---

*There are 9 practice problems scattered throughout this lesson.

FRACTIONS

The manipulation of fractions is important for the nurse because units of the Apothecaries' system are written as common fractions for all amounts less than one. Also, the nurse must be able to use an available dosage to give a dose the doctor orders when the available dose is larger or smaller than that ordered.

A *fraction* is one or more of the equal parts of a unit. The parts of the fraction are called *terms*. In the fraction $\frac{2}{3}$, the 2 and the 3 are its terms. The 2 is called the numerator and the 3 the denominator. The *denominator* tells into how many parts the whole has been divided. The *numerator* tells how many of the equal parts are taken.

Fractions are raised to higher terms by multiplying both terms of the fraction by the same number. Fractions are reduced to lower terms by dividing both the numerator and denominator by the same number. When a fraction is raised to higher terms or reduced to lower terms, the value of the fraction is not changed.

A *proper fraction* is one whose numerator is less than its denominator; eg, $\frac{3}{4}$, $\frac{1}{2}$, $\frac{1}{3}$. An *improper fraction* is one whose numerator is equal to, or greater than, its denominator; eg, $\frac{7}{7}$, $\frac{15}{3}$, $\frac{9}{2}$. An improper fraction may be changed to a whole or mixed number by dividing the numerator by the denominator.

EXAMPLE

$$\frac{15}{3} = 5, \quad \frac{9}{2} = 4\frac{1}{2}, \quad \frac{25}{5} = 5$$

A *mixed number* is composed of a whole number and a fraction: $5\frac{1}{2}$, $3\frac{1}{4}$, $1\frac{1}{2}$. To change a mixed number to an improper fraction, multiply the whole number by the denominator of the fraction and add the total to the numerator of the fraction. For example, $5\frac{1}{4}$ changed to an improper fraction is:

$$4 \times 5 = 20 + 1 = \frac{21}{4}$$

A *complex fraction* has a fraction in either its numerator or its denominator or both; for example,

$$\frac{\frac{1}{2}}{100} \quad \frac{6}{\frac{3}{4}} \quad \frac{2\frac{1}{2}}{\frac{1}{8}}$$

To change a complex fraction to a whole number, proper or improper fraction, divide the number or fraction above the line by the number or fraction below the line.

EXAMPLE: Change $\dfrac{\frac{1}{2}}{100}$ **to a proper fraction:**

$$\frac{\frac{1}{2}}{100} = \frac{1}{2} \div 100 = \frac{1}{2} \times \frac{1}{100} = \frac{1}{200}$$

SIMPLE RULES OF ARITHMETIC

Addition of Fractions

To add fractions with the same denominator, add the numerators, leave the denominator the same, and reduce to lowest terms:

$$\frac{1}{4} + \frac{1}{4} = \frac{2}{4} = \frac{1}{2}$$

To add fractions with different denominators, change to fractions having the least common denominator. The *least common denominator* is the smallest number that contains the denominator of each of the fractions a whole number of times. Divide the least common denominator by the denominator of each fraction and multiply both terms of the fraction by the quotient.

EXAMPLE

$$\frac{3}{4} + \frac{3}{8} + \frac{1}{12} + \frac{5}{6} =$$

The least common denominator of 4, 8, 12, and 6 is 24; ie, 24 is the smallest number that will yield a whole number when divided by 4, 8, 12, and 6. Thus, 24 divided by 4 = 6. Therefore, multiply both terms of the fraction by the same number.

$$\begin{array}{ll} 6 \times 3 = 18 & \dfrac{3}{4} = \dfrac{18}{24} \\ 6 \times 4 = 24 & \end{array}$$

$$\frac{3}{8} = \frac{9}{24}$$

$$\frac{1}{12} = \frac{2}{24}$$

$$\frac{5}{6} = \frac{20}{24}$$

$$\frac{49}{24} = 2\tfrac{1}{24}$$

PROBLEM 2: If the physician ordered hydromorphone hydrochloride (Dilaudid), $\frac{1}{32}$ grain, and tablets of this amount were not available, which of the following would you give?

a. 2 tablets of $\frac{1}{16}$ grain each

b. 2 tablets of $\frac{1}{64}$ grain each

Subtraction of Fractions

To subtract fractions with the same denominator, subtract the smaller numerator from the larger numerator, leave the denominators the same, and then reduce to lowest terms, if necessary.

EXAMPLE

$$\frac{7}{12} - \frac{3}{12} = \frac{4}{12} = \frac{1}{3}$$

If the fractions have different denominators, change the fractions so they will have the least common denominator (see Example, p. 10), subtract the numerator, and leave denominators the same.

EXAMPLE

$$\frac{15}{28} - \frac{3}{7} =$$

Since 28 is a multiple of 7 ($28 \div 7 = 4$), it can be used as the least common denominator. Thus,

$$3 \times 4 = 12$$
$$7 \times 4 = \overline{28}$$

The problem is then solved as follows:

$$\frac{15}{28} - \frac{12}{28} = \frac{3}{28}$$

Multiplication and Division of Fractions

1. When multiplying fractions, calculations are simplified if all possible numbers are cancelled, or divided. Denominators may be divided by numerators or vice versa to reduce them to smaller terms. After cancelling as many numbers

as possible, multiply the remaining numerators together, and then multiply the denominators.

EXAMPLE

$$\frac{1}{\cancel{100}\atop{\cancel{20}\atop 5}} \times \frac{\cancel{5}}{\cancel{6}} \times \cancel{24}^{\,\overset{1}{4}} = \frac{1}{5}$$

If the number is a mixed number, ie, a whole number and a fraction, change the number to an improper fraction and solve as below:

EXAMPLE

$$2\tfrac{1}{4} \times \frac{2}{3} \times 8 = \frac{\overset{3}{\cancel{9}}}{\cancel{4}\atop{\cancel{2}}} \times \frac{\cancel{2}}{\cancel{3}} \times \cancel{8}^{\,4} = 12$$

2. To divide a fraction by a fraction, *invert* the divisor and multiply. Cancel when possible.

EXAMPLES

$$\frac{2}{3} \div \frac{1}{3} = \frac{2}{\cancel{3}} \times \frac{\cancel{3}}{1} = 2$$

$$\frac{1}{20} \div 4 = \frac{1}{20} \times \frac{1}{4} = \frac{1}{80}$$

PROBLEM 3

$$\frac{1}{5} \times \frac{3}{4} \times 20 =$$

PROBLEM 4

$$\frac{3}{4} \div 3 =$$

Decimal Fractions

A decimal fraction is one whose denominator is 10 or some multiple of 10. Instead of writing the denominator, it is indicated by a decimal sign or decimal point (.):

$$\frac{1}{2} = 0.5$$

All numbers to the left of the decimal point represent whole numbers, and those to the right, fractions. Decimals increase in value from right to left and decrease in value left to right in multiples of 10. Zeros may be placed after the decimal point without changing the value of the whole number.

EXAMPLE

$$75 = 75. = 75.00$$

Left of Decimal Point	Right of Decimal Point
Units	Tenths
Tens	Hundredths
Hundreds	Thousandths
Thousands	Ten thousandths
Ten thousands	Hundred thousandths
Hundred thousands	Millionths

Addition and Subtraction of Decimal Fractions

To add or subtract decimal fractions, place the numbers so that the decimal points are in vertical alignment, add zeros to the right as necessary, and then add or subtract as for whole numbers. Place decimal point in answer just below the aligned decimal points in the problem.

EXAMPLE: Add the decimal fractions 0.0567 and 0.072.

$$
\begin{array}{r}
0.0567 \\
+\,0.072 \\
\hline
0.1287
\end{array}
$$

EXAMPLE: Subtract 0.02 from 0.054.

$$
\begin{array}{r}
0.054 \\
-\,0.020 \\
\hline
0.034
\end{array}
$$

Division and Multiplication of Decimal Fractions

1. To divide by a decimal fraction, first move the decimal point in the *divisor* enough places to make it a whole number. Then move the decimal point in the *dividend* as many places as it was moved in the divisor. Place the decimal point in the quotient (answer) directly above that in the dividend.

EXAMPLE: Divide 72.352 by 3.2.

$$
\begin{array}{r}
22.61 \\
3.2.\overline{)72.3.52} \\
64 \\
\hline
83 \\
64 \\
\hline
195 \\
192 \\
\hline
32 \\
32 \\
\end{array}
$$

PROBLEM 5: Divide 10.20 by 5.1.

2. To multiply decimal fractions, multiply the two numbers together and count off as many decimal places in the product (answer) as there were in the multiplier and multiplicand.

EXAMPLE

$$
\begin{array}{r}
22.61 \\
\times 3.2 \\
\hline
4522 \\
6783 \\
\hline
72.352 \\
\end{array}
$$

PROBLEM 6: Multiply 72.352 by 3.2.

Multiplication and Division by 10, 100, and 1000

1. To *multiply* a decimal fraction by 10, 100, or 1000, move the decimal point as many places to the *right* as there are whole number zeros in the multiplier.

2. To *divide* a decimal fraction by 10, 100, or 1000, move the decimal point as many places to the *left* as there are whole number zeros in the divisor.

PROBLEM 7: $0.0002 \times 1000 =$

PROBLEM 8: $0.2 \div 1000 =$

Ratio and Proportion

1. Ratio is a method of showing the relationship between two numbers and is expressed by two numbers separated by a colon. (The colon means division.) It is also another way of writing a fraction. Ratios are usually expressed in lowest terms and may be reduced by dividing both numbers by the same number.

EXAMPLE

$$50 : 100 = 1 : 2 \text{ or } \frac{1}{2}$$

This expression is read as "1 is to 2" and means there is one part to two parts; eg, in a $1 : 2$ solution, there is one part drug to two parts water or solvent.

2. Proportion is an equation between the two ratios. The first ratio equals the second. The numbers on each end are the *extremes*, and the two numbers in the middle are the *means*. *The product of the extremes equals the product of the means.* One of the terms may be an unknown (x), and the product which contains the x should be kept to the left of the equation.

EXAMPLE

$$5 : 100 :: 2 : x$$

$$5x = 200$$

$$x = 40$$

Proportions not only must be written using the same system in both ratios, but also in equal terms (metric with metric; grains with minims; and grams with cubic centimeters or milliliters).

EXAMPLE 1: If you travel 15 miles in 20 minutes, how many miles should you travel in 1 hour?

Change hours to minutes: 1 hour = 60 minutes. Then set up the proportion:

15 miles : 20 minutes = x miles : 60 minutes

Solve for x: Multiply means together = $20x$. Multiply extremes = 900.

$20x = 900$

$x = 45$ miles you should travel in 1 hour

Proportions also can be written as fractions, and cross multiplication used to solve for the unknown. Using the example above:

$$\frac{15 \text{ miles}}{20 \text{ minutes}} = \frac{x \text{ miles}}{60 \text{ minutes}}$$

Multiply the numerator of the second fraction by the denominator of the first fraction, and denominator of the second fraction by the numerator of the first fraction:

$20 \times x = 20x$ $15 \times 60 = 900$

$20x = 900$

$x = 45$ miles

EXAMPLE 2: If a solution contains 15 grains of drug to 1 quart of water, what is the ratio strength?

Grains and quarts are both in the same system (which will be discussed in Lesson 2), but are not equal terms. Milliliters and grams from the Metric system are calculated more easily, so the quart and grains should be converted to milliliters and grams.

1 quart = 1000 mL

15 grains = 1 gram

The ratio would then be 1 : 1000, or 1 g to 1000 mL.

CHANGING NUMBER FORMS

1. To change a percent to a decimal fraction, move the decimal point two places to the left and omit the percent sign. [Since percent (%) means per 100, divide by 100.]

EXAMPLE

$$25\% = 0.25 = \frac{25}{100} = \frac{1}{4} = 1 : 4$$

So 25% may be expressed as a decimal, fraction, or ratio.

NOTE: Any percent less than 1% is called a fractional percent. For example, $\frac{1}{2}$% and 0.2% are fractional percents. They are changed to common fractions and decimal fractions in the same manner as those above 1%.

EXAMPLE

a. $\frac{1}{2}\% = \dfrac{1}{2} \div 100 = \dfrac{1}{2} \times \dfrac{1}{100} = \dfrac{1}{200}$

or

$\frac{1}{2}\% = 0.5\% = 0.005$

b. $0.2\% = \dfrac{2}{10} \div 100 = \dfrac{2}{10} \times \dfrac{1}{100} = \dfrac{2}{1000} = \dfrac{1}{500}$

or

$0.2\% = 0.002$

2. To change a percent to a fraction, drop the percent sign, write the number as the numerator, 100 as the denominator, and reduce to lowest terms.

EXAMPLE

$20\% = \dfrac{20}{100} = \dfrac{1}{5}$

PROBLEM 9: Change $\frac{1}{4}$% to a fraction.

3. To change a percent to a ratio, drop the percent sign, use the number as the first term, 100 as the second term, and reduce to lowest terms; or change to a fraction and then use a colon instead of the dividing line.

EXAMPLE

$20\% = \dfrac{20}{100} = 20:100 = 1:5$

$20\% = \dfrac{20}{100} = \dfrac{1}{5} = 1:5$

4. To change a decimal fraction to a percent, move the decimal point two places to the right (multiply by 100) and add the percent sign.

EXAMPLE

$0.005 = 0.5\%$

5. To change a decimal fraction to a common fraction, omit the decimal point and place the number over the appropriate denominator of 10, 100, 1000, etc, and reduce to lowest terms.

EXAMPLE

$$0.0005 = \frac{5}{10,000} = \frac{1}{2000}$$

6. To change a decimal fraction to a ratio, write the number as the first term; then put 10, 100, 1000, etc, as the second term; finally, reduce to lowest terms.

EXAMPLE

$$0.002 = \frac{2}{1000} = \frac{1}{500} = 1:500$$

7. To change a fraction to a ratio, write the two numbers with a colon between them instead of the dividing line.

EXAMPLE

$$\frac{1}{20} = 1:20$$

8. To change a fraction to a decimal fraction, divide the numerator by the denominator.

EXAMPLE

$$\frac{1}{200} = 200\overline{)1.000}^{0.005}$$

9. To change a fraction to a percent, divide the numerator by the denominator (use as many decimal places as needed); then move the decimal point two places to the right and add the percent sign.

EXAMPLE: Change $\frac{1}{5}$ to percent.

$$5\overline{)1.00}^{0.20} = 20\%$$

10. To change a ratio to a fraction, write the numbers with a dividing line between them instead of the colon.

EXAMPLE

$$1 : 100 = \frac{1}{100}$$

11. To change a ratio to a percent, divide the first term by the second term, move the decimal point two places to the right in the answer, and add a percent sign.

EXAMPLE

$$1 : 20 = 20 \overline{)1.00} \quad \begin{array}{c} 0.05 \\ \end{array} = 5\%$$

12. To change a ratio to a decimal fraction, divide the first term by the second term.

EXAMPLE

$$1 : 20 = 20 \overline{)1.00} \quad \begin{array}{c} 0.05 \\ \end{array}$$

ANSWERS TO PROBLEMS

Problem 1

a.	XIV	b.	XLIV
c.	XLIX	d.	LXII
e.	LXXXIII	f.	XCIX

Problem 2
b is correct.

$$\frac{1}{64} + \frac{1}{64} = \frac{2}{64} = \frac{1}{32}$$

while

$$\frac{1}{16} + \frac{1}{16} = \frac{2}{16} = \frac{1}{8}$$

which is four times the dose ordered. If you answered $\frac{1}{8}$, remember to add numerators together, leave denominators the same, and reduce to lowest terms.

Problem 3

$$\frac{1}{\cancel{5}} \times \frac{3}{4} \times \cancel{20}^{\,5} = 3$$

Problem 4

$$\frac{3}{4} \div 3 = \frac{\cancel{3}^{\,1}}{4} \times \frac{1}{\cancel{3}_{\,1}} = \frac{1}{4}$$

Did you forget the rule for dividing fractions? *Invert* the divisor and multiply.

Problem 5

$$\begin{array}{r} 2. \\ 5.1\overline{)10.20} \\ \smile \\ 102 \\ \hline \end{array}$$

Answer is 2.

Problem 6
231.5264

Problem 7
Correct answer is 0.2, or did you not move the decimal point three places to the right?

Problem 8
0.0002 should be your answer. If not, review multiplication and division with multiples of 10.

Problem 9
You didn't just write $\frac{1}{4}$? Correct answer is $\frac{1}{400}$. Remember to drop the percent sign, divide by 100, and invert the divisor:

$$\tfrac{1}{4}\% = \frac{1}{4} \div 100 = \frac{1}{4} \times \frac{1}{100} = \frac{1}{400}$$

PRACTICE PROBLEMS

Write the following as Roman numerals:

1. 12 XII

2. 15 XV

3. 61 LXI

4. 75 LXXV

5. 9 IX

Write the following as Arabic numbers:

6. XLI _____

7. XXX _____

8. XVII _____

9. CDIII _____

10. XIX _____

Divide the following:

11. 50 by 0.005 _____

12. 14.4 by 0.12 _____

13. 0.15 by 0.0075 _____

14. 4.206 by 6 _____

Mentally divide each of the following numbers by 10, 100, and 1000:

15. 4.75 _____ _____ _____

16. 0.02 _____ _____ _____

17. 4 _____ _____ _____

18. 0.4 _____ _____ _____

19–22. *Mentally multiply the numbers in Problems 15 through 18 above by 10, 100, and 1000.*

Change the following to percent, decimals, fractions, and ratios:

Percent	Decimal Fraction	Fraction	Ratio
23. _____	24. _____	25. _____	26. 1 : 2
27. _____	28. _____	29. $\frac{1}{20}$	30. _____

Percent	Decimal Fraction	Fraction	Ratio
31. _____	32. 0.005	33. _____	34. _____
35. _____	36. 0.01	37. _____	38. _____
39. $\frac{1}{2}\%$	40. _____	41. _____	42. _____
43. _____	44. _____	45. $\frac{1}{4}$	46. _____
47. 2%	48. _____	49. _____	50. _____

Find the value of x *in the following ratios:*

51. $x:1000::1:5$

52. $5000:x::\dfrac{1}{10}:\dfrac{1}{2000}$

53. $x:500::\dfrac{1}{20}:2$

54. $0.0001:1::0.005:x$

Multiply the following fractions:

55. $228 \times \dfrac{1}{6}$ _____

56. $60 \times \dfrac{2}{3}$ _____

57. $\dfrac{1}{5} \times 25$ _____

58. $\dfrac{3}{10} \times 3$ _____

Multiply the following complex fractions:

59. $1\frac{7}{10} \times 2\frac{5}{8}$ _____

60. $4\frac{2}{3} \times 1\frac{1}{2}$ _____

61. $1\frac{4}{5} \times 2\frac{5}{8}$ _____

62. $8\frac{1}{4} \times 6\frac{2}{3}$ _____

Divide by fractions:

63. $4 \div \dfrac{2}{3}$ _____

64. $\dfrac{3}{5} \div \dfrac{3}{10}$ _____

65. $5 \div \dfrac{1}{5}$ _____

66. $\dfrac{1}{2} \div \dfrac{3}{4}$ _____

Divide the following complex fractions:

67. $3\frac{1}{2} \div 1\frac{3}{4}$ _____

68. $4\frac{1}{2} \div \dfrac{1}{50}$ _____

69. $2\frac{1}{2} \div 50 \times 1000$ _____

70. $40 \div 3\frac{1}{4} \times \dfrac{1}{16}$ _____

Circle the fractions with the larger value:

71. $\dfrac{5}{6}$ or $\dfrac{2}{3}$

72. $\dfrac{1}{200}$ or $\dfrac{1}{100}$

73. $\dfrac{7}{8}$ or $\dfrac{3}{4}$

74. $\dfrac{11}{12}$ or $\dfrac{7}{8}$

Arrange in order of size, from the largest to smallest value:

75. $\dfrac{9}{10}, \dfrac{4}{5}, \dfrac{17}{20}, \dfrac{3}{4}$

76. $\dfrac{1}{2}, \dfrac{9}{16}, \dfrac{17}{32}, \dfrac{5}{8}$

Circle the decimal fraction with the larger value:

77. 0.575 or 0.6

78. 0.002 or 0.0124

79. 0.725 or 0.5

80. 0.016 or 0.008

Arrange in order, from the largest to smallest value:

81. 0.54, 0.4, 0.462, 0.6145

82. 0.235, 0.024, 0.3256, 0.3

Answers to Practice Problems

1. XII	2. XV	3. LXI
4. LXXV	5. IX	
6. 41	7. 30	8. 17
9. 403	10. 19	

11. 10,000	12. 120
13. 20	14. 0.701
15. 0.475, 0.0475, 0.00475	16. 0.002, 0.0002, 0.00002
17. 0.4, 0.04, 0.004	18. 0.04, 0.004, 0.0004
19. 47.50, 475.00, 4750	20. 0.2, 2.0, 20
21. 40, 400, 4000	22. 4, 40, 400

23. 50%   24. 0.5   25. $\dfrac{1}{2}$ 26. $1:2$

27. 5%   28. 0.05   29. $\dfrac{1}{20}$ 30. 1 : 20

31. 0.5%   32. 0.005   33. $\dfrac{1}{200}$ 34. 1 : 200

35. 1%   36. 0.01   37. $\dfrac{1}{100}$ 38. 1 : 100

39. $\frac{1}{2}$%   40. 0.005   41. $\dfrac{1}{200}$ 42. 1 : 200 ($\frac{1}{2}$% is a fraction of 1%)

43. 25%   44. 0.25   45. $\dfrac{1}{4}$ 46. 1 : 4

47. 2%   48. 0.02   49. $\dfrac{1}{50}$ 50. 1 : 50

51. 200   52. 25 $5000 : x :: \dfrac{1}{10} : \dfrac{1}{2000}$

$$\frac{1}{10x} = \frac{1}{\underset{2}{\cancel{2000}}} \times \frac{\overset{5}{\cancel{5000}}}{1}$$

$$x = \frac{5}{\cancel{2}} \times \frac{\overset{5}{\cancel{10}}}{1} = 25$$

53. 12.5   54. 50
55. 38   56. 40

57. 5   58. $\dfrac{9}{10}$

59. 4.46   60. 7

61. 4.725   62. 55

63. 6   64. 2

65. 25   66. $\dfrac{2}{3}$

67. 2   68. 225

69. 50   70. $\dfrac{10}{13}$

71. $\dfrac{5}{6}$ 72. $\dfrac{1}{100}$

73. $\dfrac{7}{8}$ 74. $\dfrac{11}{12}$

75. $\dfrac{9}{10}, \dfrac{17}{20}, \dfrac{4}{5}, \dfrac{3}{4}$

$\dfrac{9}{10} = \dfrac{18}{20}$

$\dfrac{4}{5} = \dfrac{16}{20}$

$\dfrac{17}{20}$

$\dfrac{3}{4} = \dfrac{15}{20}$

76. $\dfrac{5}{8}, \dfrac{9}{16}, \dfrac{17}{32}, \dfrac{1}{2}$

77. 0.6

78. 0.0124

79. 0.725

80. 0.016

81. 0.6145, 0.54, 0.462, 0.4

82. 0.3256, 0.3, 0.235, 0.024

If you made more than nine errors, do the Additional Practice Problems with no more than eight errors before going on to Lesson 2.

ADDITIONAL PRACTICE PROBLEMS

Write the following as Roman numerals:

1. 49 _____   2. 98 _____   3. 14 _____

4. 38 _____   5. 69 _____

Write the following as Arabic numbers:

6. XLIV _____   7. XLIX _____

8. MCMLXXX _____   9. XVII _____

10. CXL _____

Divide the following:

11. 400 by 0.002 _____   12. 1000 by 2.5 _____

13. 100 by 0.5 _____   14. 2.45 by 0.2 _____

Mentally divide the following by 10, 100, *and* 1000.

15. 500 _____ _____ _____

16. 0.004 _____ _____ _____

17. 20.05 _____ _____ _____

18. 2.004 _____ _____ _____

19–22. *Mentally multiply the numbers in Problems* 15 *through* 18 *by* 10, 100, *and* 1000.

Change the following to percent, decimals, fractions, or ratios.

Percent	Decimal Fraction	Fraction	Ratio
23. _____	24. 0.02	25. _____	26. _____
27. $\frac{1}{4}\%$	28. _____	29. _____	30. _____
31. _____	32. _____	33. $\frac{1}{4}$	34. _____
35. _____	36. _____	37. _____	38. $1:20$
39. _____	40. _____	41. $\frac{1}{50}$	42. _____
43. 25%	44. _____	45. _____	46. _____

Find the value of x *in the following*:

47. $50 : x :: \frac{1}{4} : 25$　　　　48. $x : \frac{1}{4} :: \frac{1}{100} : 100$

49. $250 : x :: 5 : \frac{1}{5}$　　　　50. $\frac{1}{100} : 50 :: x : \frac{1}{5}$

Multiply the following fractions:

51. $\frac{7}{10} \times \frac{5}{8}$ _____　　　　52. $\frac{1}{8} \times \frac{4}{5}$ _____

53. $\frac{7}{8} \times \frac{1}{4}$ _____　　　　54. $15 \times \frac{4}{5}$ _____

Multiply the following complex fractions:

55. $2\frac{5}{8} \times 4\frac{2}{3}$ _____   56. $6\frac{1}{4} \times 5\frac{1}{12}$ _____

57. $7\frac{1}{2} \times 2\frac{1}{8}$ _____   58. $4\frac{1}{3} \times 2\frac{1}{6}$ _____

Divide the following fractions:

59. $\frac{4}{5}$ by 10 _____   60. $\frac{1}{100}$ by $\frac{1}{200}$ _____

61. 12 by $\frac{1}{4}$ 62. $\frac{2}{3}$ by $\frac{3}{4}$ _____

Divide the following complex fractions:

63. $\dfrac{2\frac{3}{4}}{5\frac{1}{2}}$ _____   64. $\dfrac{4\frac{1}{4}}{2\frac{1}{8}}$ _____

65. $\dfrac{3\frac{1}{3}}{50} \times 100$ _____   66. $\dfrac{20}{3\frac{1}{2}} \times \dfrac{1}{4}$ _____

Circle the fraction of larger value:

67. $\frac{3}{4}$ or $\frac{7}{8}$ 68. $\frac{5}{12}$ or $\frac{2}{3}$

69. $\frac{5}{6}$ or $\frac{3}{4}$ 70. $\frac{4}{5}$ or $\frac{2}{3}$

Arrange in order of size, from the largest to smallest value:

71. $\frac{2}{3}, \frac{3}{4}, \frac{5}{8}, \frac{5}{6}$

72. $\frac{19}{32}, \frac{9}{16}, \frac{7}{8}, \frac{3}{4}$

Circle the decimal fraction of larger value:

73. 0.324 or 0.3   74. 0.52 or 0.566

75. 0.0442 or 0.04   76. 0.016 or 0.01

Arrange in order of size, from the largest to smallest value:

77. 0.002, 0.2325, 0.2, 0.021

78. 0.5, 0.005, 0.054, 0.05

Answers to Additional Practice Problems

1. XLIX	2. XCVIII	3. XIV
4. XXXVIII	5. LXIX	
6. 44	7. 49	8. 1980
9. 17	10. 140	
11. 200,000	12. 400	
13. 200	14. 12.25	

Divide by 10	By 100	By 1000
15. 50	5	.5
16. 0.0004	0.00004	0.000004
17. 2.005	0.2005	0.02005
18. 0.2004	0.02004	0.002004

Multiply by 10	By 100	By 1000
19. 5000	50,000	500,000
20. 0.04	0.4	4.0
21. 200.5	2005	20,050
22. 20.04	200.4	20,040

23. 2%	24. 0.02	25. $\frac{1}{50}$	26. 1:50
27. $\frac{1}{4}$%	28. 0.0025	29. $\frac{1}{400}$	30. 1:400
31. 25%	32. 0.25	33. $\frac{1}{4}$	34. 1:4
35. 5%	36. 0.05	37. $\frac{1}{20}$	38. 1:20
39. 2%	40. 0.02	41. $\frac{1}{50}$	42. 1:50
43. 25%	44. 0.25	45. $\frac{1}{4}$	46. 1:4

47. 5000

48. $\dfrac{1}{40,000}$

49. 10

50. $\dfrac{1}{25,000}$

51. $\dfrac{7}{16}$

52. $\dfrac{1}{10}$

53. $\dfrac{7}{32}$

54. 12

55. $12\frac{1}{4}$

56. 31.77

57. 15.93

58. 9.38

59. $\dfrac{2}{25}$

60. 2

61. 48

62. $\dfrac{8}{9}$

63. $\dfrac{1}{2}$

64. 2

65. $6\frac{2}{3}$

66. $1\frac{3}{7}$

67. $\dfrac{7}{8}$

68. $\dfrac{2}{3}$

69. $\dfrac{5}{6}$

70. $\dfrac{4}{5}$

71. $\dfrac{5}{6}, \dfrac{3}{4}, \dfrac{2}{3}, \dfrac{5}{8}$

72. $\dfrac{7}{8}, \dfrac{3}{4}, \dfrac{19}{32}, \dfrac{9}{16}$

73. 0.324

74. 0.566

75. 0.0442

76. 0.016

77. 0.2325, 0.2, 0.021, 0.002

78. 0.5, 0.054, 0.05, 0.005

LESSON 2

Apothecaries' and Metric Systems of Weights and Measures

Objectives

After completing this lesson, the student will be able to:

- Demonstrate an understanding of the Apothecaries' system by changing from one measure to another in that system.

- Demonstrate an understanding of the Metric system by changing from one measure to another in that system.

- Compare the units used in the Apothecaries' and Metric systems.

- Identify the abbreviations used to express units in both systems.

- Identify common abbreviations and symbols that are used in this text as given on page 213, Appendix D.

- Solve the practice problems at the end of this lesson with no more than five errors.

The systems of weights and measures commonly used in the preparation of drugs are the Apothecaries' (England) and the Metric (France) or decimal system. Household measures are approximate measures that are used only when more accurate measures are not available. Teaspoons, tablespoons, cups, glasses, or tumblers are household measures.

Because the U.S. government's goal to convert entirely to the Metric system by 1983 was not accomplished, it is necessary to have a thorough knowledge of both systems in order to administer drugs or prepare solutions accurately, safely, and quickly. (See Appendix A, Rules for Giving Medications.)

THE METRIC SYSTEM

The *meter* is the fundamental unit of the Metric system (Table 1). It is from this standard linear measure that the other two Metric units of weight and volume are derived.

The Metric unit of capacity or volume is the *liter*. It was decided that the standard for volume would be a cube measuring exactly 1 decimeter (10 times as large as a centimeter) in length on all sides, and, when this container was filled, the volume it held would equal exactly 1 liter.

The *milliliter* is the division of the liter most commonly used in hospitals, and since 1000 cubes measuring 1 centimeter on all sides equal a liter, then 1000 cubic centimeters also equals a liter; therefore, 1 cc = 1 mL. (Since a milliliter is 0.001 of a liter, there are 1000 mL in a liter.)

The *kilogram*, which weighs approximately 2.2 pounds, is also used frequently in hospitals to express *weight*. The kilogram proved to be too large to

TABLE 1. THE METRIC SYSTEM

Solid Measure	Volume or Liquid Measure
1000 micrograms (µg) = 1 milligram (mg)	1000 cubic centimeters (cc)
1000 milligrams = 1 gram (g)*	or
1000 grams = 1 kilogram (kg)	1000 milliliters (mL)† = 1 liter (L)

Note: Cubic centimeters, milliliters, and grams are equivalent, since 1 cc or 1 mL weighs approximately 1 g. Kilograms are used frequently to determine dosage by weight.

$$1 \text{ cc} = 1 \text{ mL} = 1 \text{ g}$$
$$1 \text{ kg} = 2.2 \text{ lb}$$

Since 1000 mg equals 1 g and 1000 micrograms (µg) = 1 milligram:

To change milligrams to grams: Move the decimal point three places to the *left* (divide by 1000).

To change grams to milligrams: Move the decimal point three places to the *right* (multiply by 1000).

To change micrograms to milligrams: Move decimal point three places to the *left*.

To change milligrams to microgram: Move decimal point three places to *right*.

---

*Gram is here abbreviated with the lower-case letter (g). To avoid confusion, grain should not be abbreviated. The student may find gram also abbreviated as gm in other texts.

†Although the abbreviation for milliliter is expressed as ml in most textbooks, mL will be used in this text as it is the abbreviation adopted by the American Medical Association.

meet the needs of pharmacists, so the *gram* was chosen as their basic unit of *weight*. The gram is 0.001 of a kilogram; therefore, there are 1000 g in 1 kg.

Fractional parts of a gram are expressed in *milligrams*. Since *milli-* signifies a thousandth (0.001), then 1000 mg = 1 g.

> 1 cc = 1 mL and weighs 1 g
> 1 kg = 2.2 lbs

Grams and milligrams are Metric drug *weights*, or solid measure; therefore, answers to dosage problems (drugs for injection) should be in milliliters, or cubic centimeters (fluid measures) rather than in milligrams, or grams.

The prefixes of the Metric system used to indicate multiples or fractions of a unit commonly used in hospitals are *kilo-* (kilogram), which indicates 1000 times the unit (gram); *centi-*, which indicates the hundredth (0.01) part of a unit (centimeter); and *milli-*, which represents the thousandth (0.001) part of a unit (milligram).

THE APOTHECARIES' SYSTEM

In the Apothecaries' system (Table 2) the units used are the grain and minim. Arabic symbols are used to denote some of the units (ʒ for dram and ʒ for ounce*), and lower-case Roman numerals are usually used to express quantity: i,

TABLE 2. THE APOTHECARIES' SYSTEM*

Solid Measure	Liquid Measure
60 grains = 1 dram (dr or ʒ)	60 minims (*m*) = 1 fluid dram (fʒ)
8 drams = 1 ounce (oz or ʒ)	8 fluid drams = 1 fluid ounce (f ʒ or fl oz)
480 grains = 1 ounce	
12 ounces = 1 pound (lb)†	16 fluid ounces = 1 pint (pt or O.)
	2 pints = 1 quart (qt)
	4 quarts = 1 gallon (gal)
	480 minims = 1 ounce

Note: Minims and grains are equivalent, since 1 minim weighs approximately 1 grain.

*Only those units most commonly used are given.
†Note that in the Apothecaries' and Troy tables 12 oz = 1 lb generally is not used by nurses, while 16 oz = 1 lb in the Avoirdupois table is used commonly.

*The student may also find the symbol *m* used to represent the Apothecaries' minim. This should not be confused with the Metric "m" for meter.

v, cx, etc. However, when fractional quantities are required, Arabic numbers are used, although the special abbreviation, *ss* (Latin, *semis*), can be used in place of $\frac{1}{2}$. Note that when using an Apothecary abbreviation the unit precedes the quantity.

EXAMPLE

$$\mathfrak{z}\,\text{iii, grains x,} \quad \frac{3}{4}\,\text{, grains}\,\frac{1}{2}\,\text{, grains iss}\left(1\tfrac{1}{2}\right).$$

If the unit is not abbreviated, the amount is written in Arabic numbers before the unit, eg, 4 grains.

The units in the Apothecaries' system for weighing drugs are grain, dram, ounce, and pound. The units for measuring liquids are minim, dram (fluid dram), ounce, pint, quart, and gallon.

1 minim weighs 1 grain

Most problems are solved more efficiently using the Metric system. Therefore, it is advisable to convert units in the Apothecaries' system to the Metric system, especially when large amounts are involved.

In converting from the Apothecaries' system to the Metric system, or even when working problems using only the Apothecaries' system, equivalents are used that are not exactly correct, but have been found to be accurate enough for all practical purposes. (Units in the Apothecaries' system are not exactly equal to equivalent units in the Metric system.) For example, 500 minims or 500 grains to the ounce may be used instead of 480 minims or 480 grains, but only when 1 to 3 oz are involved. Another example is in the conversion of grains to grams, or grams to grains. There is a slight discrepancy in the results. For example, 0.016 g equals 0.24 grain, but since dosage in Apothecaries' is written as *small* common fractions, 0.24 is reduced to the *nearest, smallest fraction* by dividing the numerator into the denominator and obtaining the nearest whole number as an answer: $0.24 = \frac{24}{100} = \frac{1}{4}$.

"Rounding off" is acceptable only in a few situations. Generally, if your answer in minims is less than $\frac{1}{2}$, or more than $\frac{1}{2}$, you may round off. For example, if your answer is $8\frac{1}{5}$ *m*, you would give 8 *m*; but if the answer is $8\frac{3}{4}$ *m*, you would give 9 *m*. It is *not* acceptable to round off milliliters, pediatric and neonatal dosage, medications for diagnostic tests, tablets, capsules, insulin, or cardiotonics.

COMPARISON OF METRIC AND APOTHECARIES' SYSTEMS

Metric System	**Apothecaries' System**
Common units: milligram, gram, cubic centimeter, milliliter, and liter.	Common units: grain, minim, dram, and ounce.
Arabic numbers and decimal fractions are used.	Roman numerals and common fractions are used.
The number is *followed* by the abbreviation.	Abbreviations or symbols *precede* the number.
Example: morphine 0.016 g.	*Example*: morphine grains $\frac{1}{4}$.

COMMON ABBREVIATIONS

Abbreviation	Latin Derivations	Meaning
@		at
aa	*ana*	of each
ac	*ante cibum*	before meals
ad lib	*ad libitum*	as desired
bid	*bis in die*	twice a day
$\bar{c}$		with
cap		capsule
dr		dram
elix		elixir
g		gram
grain		grain
guttae	*guttae*	drop
(H)		hypodermically
hs	*hora somni*	at bedtime
IM		intramuscular
IV		intravenous
kg		kilogram
m		minim
mEq		milliequivalents
od	*oculus dexter*	right eye
oh	*omni hora*	every hour
om	*omni mane*	every morning
on	*omni nocte*	every night

os	*oculus sinister*	left eye
os	*os*	mouth
ou	*oculus uterque*	each eye
oz		ounce
pc	*post cibum*	after meals
prn	*pro re nata*	according to necessity
qd	*quaque die*	every day
qhr	*quaque hora*	every hour
qid	*quator in die*	four times a day
qs	*quantum sufficit*	quantity sufficient
s̄		without
sc		subcutaneous
sol		solution
sos	*si opus sit*	administer once if necessary
ss	*semis*	one-half
stat	*statim*	at once
tid	*ter in die*	three times a day

PRACTICE PROBLEMS

1. List the five common units used in the Metric system.

2. List the four common units used in the Apothecaries' system.

Give abbreviations for the following:

3. grain _____   4. gram _____

5. kilogram _____   6. dram _____

7. milligram _____   8. cubic centimeter _____

9. minim _____   10. ounce _____

11. In the Apothecaries' system (*numbers, numerals*) are used. The abbreviation or symbol (*precedes, follows*) the quantity.

12. Common fractions are used in the _____ system and follow the symbol or abbreviation.

13. Atropine 0.4 mg is written in the _____ system.

14. Sulfasuxidine grain xv is written in the _____ system.

Make the following conversions between the Metric and Apothecaries' systems:

2.2 lb = 1000 g = 1 kg   454 g = 1 lb

15. 2500 g = __1__ kg = _____ lb

16. 7½ lb = _____ kg = _____ g

17. 115 lb = _____ kg

18. 40 kg = _____ lb = _____ g

19. 2.2 lb = _____ kg = _____ g

20. 1 mg = _____ μg (microgram)

21. 100 μg = _____ mg

22. 0.2 mg = _____ μg

Convert the following:

23. 180 grains = _____ dram (℈)

24. $\frac{1}{4}$ dram = _____ grains

25. $\frac{1}{2}$ dram = _____ grains

26. ℥iv = _____ ounce (℥)

Convert the following:

27. ℥ii (2 oz) = _____ drams

28. ℥vi = _____ drams

29. 1 pt = _____ quart

30. 1 oz = _____ drams

Give the Metric equivalents for the following:

31. 1 kg = _____ g

32. 1 mg = _____ g

33. 1 g = _____ mg

34. 0.4 mg = _____ g

35. 0.0032 g = _____ mg

Give the Metric equivalents for the following:

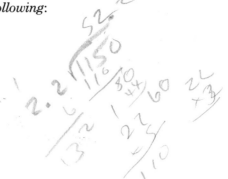

36. 1 mL = ___1___ cc

37. 1 liter = __1000__ mL

38. 50 mL = __.05__ liter

39. 100 cc = __100__ mL

40. 500 mL = __.5__ liter

Answers to Practice Problems

1. Common units in Metric system are:
   a. milligram (mg)
   b. gram (g)
   c. cubic centimeter (cc)
   d. milliliter (mL)
   e. liter (L)
2. Common units in Apothecaries' system are:
   a. grain
   b. minim (*m*)
   c. dram (dr or ℥)
   d. ounce (oz or ℥)

3. grain (do not abbreviate)
5. kg
7. mg
9. *m*

4. g
6. dr or ℥
8. cc
10. oz or ℥

11. Roman numerals, precedes
12. Apothecaries'
13. Metric
14. Apothecaries'
15. 2.5 kg, 5.5 lb
16. 3.4 kg, 3400 g
17. 52 kg
18. 88 lb, 40,000 g
19. 1 kg, 1000 g
20. 1 mg = 1000 μg

21. 100 µg = 0.1 mg
22. 0.2 mg = 200 µg
23. 3 drams (℥ iii)
24. 15 grains
25. 30 grains (grain xxx)
26. $\frac{1}{2}$ oz (℥ ss)
27. 16 drams (℥ xvi)
28. 48 drams (℥ xlviii)
29. $\frac{1}{2}$ quart
30. 8 drams (℥ viii)
31. 1000 g
32. 0.001 g
33. 1000 mg
34. 0.0004 g
35. 3.2 mg
36. 1 cc
37. 1000 mL
38. 0.05 liter
39. 100 mL
40. 0.5 liter

If you made no more than five errors, go on to Lesson 3. If not, do the Additional Practice Problems with no more than six errors before proceeding.

ADDITIONAL PRACTICE PROBLEMS

1. Grams and cubic centimeter are units of the _____ system.

2. Minim is a unit of measure in the _____ system.

Give abbreviations for the following:

3. quart _____   4. liter _____   5. pint _____

6. milliliter _____   7. dram _____   8. ounce _____

Indicate to which system of measurement each of the following belongs—Metric (*M*), *Apothecaries' (A):*

9. g _____   10. cc _____   11. mL _____

12. grains _____   13. liter _____   14. pt _____

15. minims _____   16. mg _____   17. ℥ _____

18. ℥ _____

19. State the rule for changing grams to milligrams and milligrams to grams.

Give the equivalents for the following amounts in the Apothecaries' system:

20. ~~grains~~ lx = _____ dram   21. grains xv = _____ minims

22. *m* xxx = _____ dram   23. grains xxx = __½__ dram

24. grains 240 = __⅛__ ounce   25. ℥ ii = __120__ grain

26. ℥ ss = __4__ dram   27. 1 lb = _____ oz

Give the equivalents for the following amounts in the Metric system:

28. 0.5 g = __500__ mg   29. 1 liter = __1000__ cc

30. 1 liter = __1000__ mL   31. 100 mg = __.1__ g

32. 1 kg = __1000__ g   33. 0.005 g = _____ mg

34. 1000 μg = __1__ mg   35. 500 mL = _____ liter

36. 500 mg = _____ g   37. 0.0004 g = _____ mg

38. 150 mg = _____ g   39. 1400 g = _____ kg

40. 3 kg = _____ g   41. 0.04 g = _____ mg

42. 1200 mg = _____ g

43. 1.5 liter = __1500__ mL   44. 0.5 liter = __500__ cc

45. 3000 mL = _____ liter   46. 0.25 liter = _____ cc

47. 4500 g = _____ kg = _____ lb

48. 6 lb = _____ g = _____ kg

49. 1 kg = _____ g = _____ lb

50. 100 lb = _____ kg = _____ g

51. 2000 g = _____ kg = _____ lb

Answers to Additional Practice Problems

1. Metric
2. Apothecaries'

3. qt	4. L	5. pt
6. mL	7. dr or ʒ	8. oz or ʒ
9. M	10. M	11. M
12. A	13. M	14. A
15. A	16. M	17. A
18. A		

19. *Milli-* means thousandths; therefore, 1000 mg = 1 g. Thus, you would *multiply* to change grams to milligrams, or move the decimal point three places to the *right*. To change milligrams to grams, move the decimal point three places to the *left* (divide).

20. ʒ i	21. *m* xv	22. ʒ ss
23. ʒ ss	24. ʒ ss	25. 120 grains
26. ʒ iv	27. 12 oz or ʒ xii	
28. 500 mg	29. 1000 cc	30. 1000 mL
31. 0.1 g	32. 1000 g	33. 5 mg
34. 1 mg	35. 0.5 liter	36. 0.5 g
37. 0.4 mg		
38. 0.15 g	39. 1.4 kg	40. 3000 g
41. 40 mg	42. 1.2 g	
43. 1500 mL		44. 500 mL
45. 3 liters		46. 250 cc

47. 4.5 kg, 9.9 lb
48. 2724 g, 2.7 kg
49. 1000 g, 2.2 lb
50. 45.4 kg, 45,400 g
51. 2 kg, 4.4 lb

LESSON 3

Metric and Apothecaries' Equivalents

Objectives

After completing this lesson, and without referring to a book, the student will be able to:

- List selected Metric–Apothecaries' equivalents.

- Demonstrate an understanding of Metric–Apothecaries' equivalents by changing:
  a. Grams to grains
  b. Grains to grams
  c. Grains to milligrams
  d. Milligrams to grains
  e. Milligrams to grams
  f. Grams to milligrams.

- Solve the practice problems at the end of this lesson with no more than six errors.

METRIC AND APOTHECARIES' SYSTEMS EQUIVALENTS

The student should become familiar with the following equivalent values in the two systems of measurement:

Metric System		**Apothecaries' System**
1 mg	=	$\frac{1}{60}$ grain
60 or 64 mg* or 0.06 g	=	1 grain
1 g, 1 mL, or 1 cc	=	15–16 grains, 15–16 minims
4–5 g or 4–5 mL or 4–5 cc	=	1 dram, 60–64 grains, 60–64 minims
30–32 g, 30–32 cc, 30–32 mL	=	1 oz, 8 drams
500 g, 500 mL, 500 cc	=	1 pt or 16 oz
1 liter, 1000 mL, 1000 cc	=	1 qt
1000 g or 1 kg	=	2.2 lb
4000 cc, 4000 mL, 4 liters	=	1 gal

NOTE: There are actually 64 mg in 1 grain and 16 grains in 1 g, but since 60 and 15 are easier to make calculations, they may be employed in making conversions.

Remember:

---
60 or 64 mg = 1 grain
15–16 grain = 1 g
1000 mg = 1 g

RULES FOR CONVERTING

To Change:	**Method:**
Grams to grains or milliliters to minims:	Multiply by 15 or 16.[†]
Grains to grams or minims to cubic centimeters:	Divide by 15 or 16.[†]

---

*The *U.S. Pharmacopeia* also lists 65 and 66.6 mg = 1 grain.

[†]See note at top of page 45.

To Change:	Method:
Grains to milligrams:	Multiply by 60 or 64.
Milligrams to grains:	Divide by 60 or 64.
Milligrams to grams:	Move decimal point three places to *left*. (Divide by 1000, since 1000 mg = 1 g.)
Grams to milligrams:	Move decimal point three places to the *right*. (Multiply by 1000.)

NOTE: When grams are converted to grains or grains are converted to grams, the result is a large fraction that is difficult to reduce. Therefore, it is easier to first convert the grams to milligrams by moving the decimal point three places to the right, and then dividing by 60 or 64 to convert the milligrams to grains.

EXAMPLE: Change 0.008 g to grains.

Move the decimal point three places to the right:

$$0.008 \text{ g} = 8 \text{ mg} \div 64 = \frac{8}{64} = \text{grain } \frac{1}{8}$$

In contrast, if you multiply 0.008 by 16 in order to change grams to grains, the result is a large decimal fraction which has to be changed to a regular fraction and then reduced.

EXAMPLE

$$0.008 \times 16 = 0.128 = \frac{128}{1000} = \frac{1}{8}$$

When converting grains to grams, multiply by 60 or 64; ie, change to milligrams first, and then move the decimal point three places to the left.

EXAMPLE: Change grain $\frac{1}{100}$ to grams.

First, convert the grains to milligrams:

$$\text{grain } \frac{1}{100} \times 60 = \frac{60}{100} = \frac{6}{10} = 0.6 \text{ mg}$$

Then convert milligrams to grams by moving the decimal point three places to the left:

0.6 mg = 0.0006 g (divide by 1000)

In contrast, converting grain $\frac{1}{100}$ directly to grams by dividing by 15 requires the following operations:

$$\text{grains } \frac{1}{100} \div 15 = \frac{1}{100} \times \frac{1}{15} = \frac{1}{1500} = 1500 \overline{)1.0000} \ ^{0.0006 \text{ g}}$$

As stated previously, work problems by the method that *you* understand best and that is easiest for *you*.

Examples of Converting Between Systems

EXAMPLE: Change 0.016 g to grains.

The easiest method to convert grains to grams or grams to grains is to change either to milligrams first. So 0.016 g = 16 mg (move decimal point 3 places to right); then divide by 64 (there being 64 mg in 1 grain):

$$16 \div 64 = \frac{16}{64} = \frac{1}{4} \text{ so, } 0.016 \text{ g} = \text{grain } \frac{1}{4}$$

Or, you may change grams to grains by multiplying by 15; however this method is not recommended as there are more chances for error.

0.016 g × 15 = 0.24 grain

But since grains are written as small common fractions, 0.24 must be changed to a small fraction:

$$0.24 = \frac{24}{100} = \frac{1}{4}$$

(rounding off $\frac{24}{100}$ to the smallest equivalent fraction with one for a numerator by dividing the denominator by the numerator.)

EXAMPLE: Change grain $\frac{1}{16}$ to grams.

To change grains to grams, first change to milligrams by multiplying by 64:

$$\frac{1}{\cancel{16}} \times \overset{4}{\cancel{64}} = 4 \, \text{mg}$$

Then move the decimal point three places to the left:

4 mg = 0.004 g

Or, to change grains to grams divide by 15:

$$\frac{1}{16} \div 15 = \frac{1}{16} \times \frac{1}{15} = \frac{1}{240}$$

But since grams are expressed as decimals, the fraction must be changed:

$$240\overline{)1.000}^{\,0.004 \, \text{g}} \quad \text{Thus, grain } \tfrac{1}{16} = 0.004 \text{ g.}$$

EXAMPLE: Change grain $\frac{1}{4}$ to milligrams.

To change grains to mg, multiply by 60 or 64:

$$\frac{1}{\cancel{4}} \times \overset{16}{\cancel{64}} = 16 \, \text{mg}$$

EXAMPLE: Change 100 mg to grains.

To change milligrams to grains, divide by 60 or 64:

100 ÷ 64 = 1.5

The answer would then be expressed as grain $1\frac{1}{2}$.

Points to Remember

1. Work problems the *easy* way. Generally it is easier to convert grams to grains or milligrams when these units are in a problem.

2. If two systems are involved in determining equivalents, eg, mg, g (Metric), and grains (Apothecaries'), first convert using the same system, ie, g to mg (Metric) or vice versa, and *then* to grains using whichever unit is easier to convert.

EXAMPLE: grain $\frac{1}{4}$ = _____ **g =** _____ **mg**

In this example it is easier to convert grains to milligrams ($\frac{1}{4} \times 64 = 16$ mg) and then to convert 16 mg to grams by moving the decimal point three places to the left, rather than changing grain $\frac{1}{4}$ to grams:

$$\frac{1}{4} \div 15 = \frac{1}{4} \times \frac{1}{15} = \frac{1}{60} = 0.016 \text{ g}$$

NOTE: Decimal fractions should be used with grams and milligrams.

EXAMPLE 2: 0.5 g = _____ **grains =** _____ **mg**

First, convert 0.5 g to mg by moving the decimal point three places to the right (= 500 mg) and *then* convert to grains using the simplest method.
    a. 0.5 g $\times$ 15 = grain $7\frac{1}{2}$ (grain viiss)
    b. 500 mg $\div$ 60 = grain $7\frac{1}{2}$

EXAMPLE 3: 1000 mg = _____ **grains =** _____ **g**

The answers can be found from the list of equivalents (p. 44) and should be so stated: 15–16 grains, 1 g.
    3. If you can solve your problems mentally, do not calculate on paper.
    4. Fractions of dosage in grains are written almost always in *small* fractions with one for a numerator. Therefore, reduce fractions to lowest terms by dividing the denominator by the numerator.

EXAMPLE: Give 0.01 g morphine from grain $\frac{1}{4}$.

$$0.01 \text{ g} \times 15 \text{ grains} = 0.15 = \frac{15}{100} = \text{grain}\frac{1}{6}$$

    5. When dividing fractions, invert the divisor before multiplying:

$$\frac{1}{4} \div 2 = \frac{1}{4} \times \frac{1}{2} = \frac{1}{8}$$

    6. When multiplying fractions, cancel as many numbers as possible before multiplying:

$$\frac{1}{\underset{1}{4}} \times \frac{\overset{2}{\cancel{8}}}{\underset{3}{\cancel{9}}} \times \frac{\overset{1}{\cancel{3}}}{\underset{2}{\cancel{4}}} = \frac{1}{6}$$

7. Solve problems logically, and not from memorization. *You do have to memorize your equivalent tables.*

EXAMPLE: Change 100 mg to grams.

If you remember that 1000 mg = 1 g, then you should know that 100 mg will not be 100,000 g. If there is any doubt as to whether you should multiply or divide, write your equivalents down and place whatever you are trying to find just below it. This should help you to see whether your answer will be larger or smaller.

1000 mg = 1 g

100 mg = ____ g

100 mg = 0.1 g

This will show you that you should divide.

8. In fractions, the denominator denotes the number of parts into which the whole has been divided. Therefore, the larger the denominator, the *smaller* the value of each part of the fraction because there are more parts of the whole. For example, would you rather have a slice of pie from one that has been cut into 16 pieces ($\frac{1}{16}$) or from one that has been cut into 6 pieces ($\frac{1}{6}$)?

9. It is advisable to work problems by more than one formula or method to double check your answers.

10. Dosage for different drugs falls within a short range of closely related fractions, or decimal fractions, as shown in the examples below

Drug	Metric System	Apothecaries' System
Morphine	0.016, 0.01, 0.008 g or 16, 10, 8 mg	grains $\frac{1}{4}, \frac{1}{6}, \frac{1}{8}$
Omnopon	20, 10 mg	grains $\frac{1}{3}, \frac{1}{6}$
Codeine	64, 32, 16 mg	grains i, $\frac{1}{2}, \frac{1}{4}$
Atropine	0.6, 0.4, 0.3 mg	grains $\frac{1}{100}, \frac{1}{150}, \frac{1}{200}$

If for example you are preparing an injection of atropine grain $\frac{1}{150}$ and your answer is grain $\frac{1}{6}$, by looking at the table you should know that you have made an error since the amounts do not vary that much.

NOTE: Although there are a few exceptions, most of the fractions used to express the amount in grains have a numerator of 1.

PRACTICE PROBLEMS

Give the Apothecaries' equivalent for the following:

1. 1 mg $\frac{1}{60}$ gr   2. 1 kg 2.2 lb   3. 1 liter 1 qt

4. 1 g 15 gr   5. 500 cc 1 pint

Convert grams to grains (show your work):

6. 15 g = grain 225   7. 1 g = grain 15

8. 0.5 g = grain 7.5   9. 0.016 g = grain 1/4

10. 0.01 g = grain .15

Convert grains to grams:

11. grain xv = ___1___ g   12. grain iii = __.2__ g

13. grain $\frac{1}{2}$ = __.03__ g   14. grain $\frac{1}{32}$ = _____ g

15. grain viiss = __.5__ g

Convert grains to milligrams:

16. grain $\frac{1}{6}$ = __10__ mg   17. grain $\frac{1}{10}$ = __6__ mg

18. grain ii = __120__ mg   19. grain vi = __360__ mg

20. grain $\frac{1}{100}$ = __.6__ mg

Convert milligrams to grains:

21. 60 mg = grain __1__   22. 5 mg = grain __1/12__

23. 15 mg = grain __1/4__   24. 0.4 mg = grain __1/150__

25. 1 mg = grain _____

Convert milligrams to grams:

26. 1000 mg = _____ g   27. 10 mg = _____ g

28. 60 mg = _____ g   29. 0.4 mg = _____ g

30. 0.1 mg = _____ g

Convert grams to milligrams:

31. 1 g = _____ mg   32. 0.06 g = _____ mg

33. 0.065 g = _____ mg   34. 0.0004 g = _____ mg

35. 0.016 g = _____ mg

Give the Metric equivalent for the following:

36. 1 oz = _____   37. 1 dram = _____   38. 1 grain = _____

39. 1 gal = _____   40. 1 qt = _____

41. If the physician orders 2 g of sulfadiazine initially, then 1 g every 6 hours for 72 hours, how many tablets would you order for the 72-hour supply if each tablet is 0.5 g each?

42. 1 pint = _____ cc

43. 60 cc = _____ oz

Convert the following:

44. grain xv = _____ g = _____ mg

45. 0.01 g = grain _____ = _____ mg

46. 16 mg = grain _____ = _____ g

47. 0.4 mg = _____ g = grain _____

48. 0.008 g = _____ mg = grain _____

Answers to Practice Problems

1. grain $\dfrac{1}{60}$ 2. 1 qt or 2.2 lb   3. 1 qt

4. 15–16 grains   5. 1 pt

6. 225 grains [Did you multiply or divide? Remember, 15 grains = 1 g]

7. grain xv   8. grain viiss

9. grain $\dfrac{1}{4}$ 10. grain $\dfrac{1}{6}$

11. 1 g   12. 0.2 g   13. 0.03 g

14. 0.002 g   15. 0.5 g

16. 10 mg   17. 6 mg   18. 120 mg

19. 360 mg   20. 0.6 mg

21. grain i   22. grain $\dfrac{1}{12}$ 23. grain $\dfrac{1}{4}$

24. grain $\dfrac{1}{150}$ 25. grain $\dfrac{1}{60}$

26. 1 g   27. 0.01 g   28. 0.06 g

29. 0.0004 g   30. 0.0001 g

31. 1000 mg   32. 60 mg   33. 65 mg

34. 0.4 mg   35. 16 mg

36. 30 g or 30 cc or 30 mL   37. 4 g, 4 cc, 4 mL

38. 60 mg, 64 mg, 0.06 g   39. 4000 cc or 4 liters

40. 1000 cc or 1 liter

41. 28 tablets. 2 g initially, or 4 tablets (0.5 g each) plus 1 g, or 2 tablets, every 6 hours for 72 hours would be 12 doses. Thus, 4 + 24 (2 × 12) = 28 tablets.

42. 500 cc

43. 2 oz or ℥ ii

44. 1 g, 1000 mg

45. grain $\dfrac{1}{6}$, 10 mg [It would be easier to convert g to mg and then convert to grains.]

46. grain $\dfrac{1}{4}$, 0.016 g   47. 0.0004 g, grain $\dfrac{1}{150}$

48. 8 mg, grain $\dfrac{1}{8}$

If you made no more than six errors, go on to Lesson 4. If not, solve the Additional Practice Problems with no more than six errors before proceeding.

ADDITIONAL PRACTICE PROBLEMS

Give the Apothecaries' equivalent for the following:

1. 1 mL _15 minims_   2. 60 mg _gr_   3. 30 cc _1 oz_

4. 1000 cc _1 qt_   5. 4 mL _1 dram_

Give Metric equivalent for the following:

6. 1 pt _500 cc_   7. $\mathfrak{z}$ viii _240_   8. grain lx _____

9. grain $\frac{1}{60}$ _1 mg_   10. m 60 _4 cc_

Convert grams to grains:

11. 0.001 g = grain _.015_   12. 0.1 g = grain _1.5_

13. 0.65 g = grain _____   14. 0.02 g = grain _.3_

15. 0.0003 g = grain _____

Convert grains to grams:

16. grain x = _.6_ g   17. grain $\frac{1}{6}$ = _.01_ g

18. grain $\frac{1}{64}$ = _____ g   19. grain $\frac{3}{4}$ = _____ g

20. grain $\frac{1}{100}$ = _____ g

Convert grains to milligrams:

21. grain $\frac{1}{4}$ = _____ mg   22. grain ss = _____ mg

23. grain ii = _____ mg   24. grain $\frac{1}{32}$ = _____ mg

25. grain $\frac{1}{150}$ = _____ mg

Convert milligrams to grains:

26. 300 mg = grain _5_   27. 10 mg = grain _____

28. 1.6 mg = grain _____   29. 0.6 mg = grain _____

30. 0.3 mg = grain _____

Convert milligrams to grams:

31. 32 mg = _____ g   32. 16 mg = _____ g

33. 0.6 mg = _____ g   34. 48 mg = _____ g

35. 8 mg = _____ g

Convert grams to milligrams:

36. 2 g = _____ mg   37. 0.006 g = _____ mg

38. 0.003 g = _____ mg   39. 0.01 g = _____ mg

40. 0.1 g = _____ mg   41. 1 gallon = _____ ml

42. 1 quart = _____ cc

Convert the following quantities:

43. grain viiss = _____ mg = _____ g

44. 0.3 g = grain _____ = _____ mg

45. 10 mg = _____ g = grain _____

46. grain v = _____ g = _____ mg

47. 0.3 mg = grain _____ = _____ g

Answers to Additional Practice Problems

1. 15 or 16 minims

2. 1 grain

3. 1 oz

4. 1 qt

5. 1 dram

6. 500 cc

7. 30–32 cc or 30–32 g

8. 4 g or 4 mL or 4 cc

9. 1 mg

10. 4 mL or 4 cc or 4 g

11. grain $\dfrac{1}{60}$

12. grain iss

13. grain x (This is an example of the discrepancy when changing from one system to another as 0.65 g × 15 = 9.75, which should be rounded to 10 grains.)

14. grain $\dfrac{1}{3}$

15. grain $\dfrac{1}{200}$

16. 0.6 g

17. 0.01 g

18. 0.001 g

19. 0.045 g

20. 0.0006 g

21. 16 mg

22. 32 mg

23. 120 mg

24. 2 mg

25. 0.4 mg

26. grain v

27. grain $\dfrac{1}{6}$

28. grain $\dfrac{1}{40}$

29. grain $\dfrac{1}{100}$

30. grain $\dfrac{1}{200}$

31. 0.032 g

32. 0.016 g

33. 0.0006 g

34. 0.048 g

35. 0.008 g

36. 2000 mg

37. 6 mg

38. 3 mg

39. 10 mg

40. 100 mg

41. 4000 mL

42. 1000 cc

43. 500 mg, 0.5 g

44. grain v, 300 mg

45. 0.01 g, grain $\dfrac{1}{6}$

46. 0.3 g, 300 mg

47. grain $\dfrac{1}{200}$, 0.0003 g

LESSON 4

Household Measures and their Equivalents

Objectives

After completing this lesson, the student will be able to:

- List the common household measures.

- Identify abbreviations for common household measures.

- Identify equivalents for the systems of Apothecaries', Metric, and household measures.

- Solve the practice problems with no more than four errors without referring to a book.

Household measures (Table 3) are used primarily in the home for measuring liquids when other measures are not available. They are approximate measures and should not be used when other measures are available. They should never be used to measure potent drugs.

The *equivalent* units for household measures in the Apothecaries' and Metric systems are shown below (see also Figs. 1 and 2).

TABLE 3. SUMMARY OF HOUSEHOLD MEASURES

60 drops (guttae) = 1 teaspoonful (t; also tsp)
4 teaspoonsful = 1 tablespoonful (T; also Tbs)
2 tablespoonsful = 1 ounce (oz)
6 ounces = 1 teacupful
8 ounces = 1 glassful or 1 tumblerful
8 teaspoonsful = 1 ounce

Household Measures	Apothecaries' System	Metric System
1 teaspoonful	1 dram or 60 minims	4 or 5 cc*
1 tablespoonful	3 or 4 drams	15 or 16 cc
2 tablespoonsful	8 drams or 1 ounce	30 or 32 cc*
1 teacupful	6 ounces	180 cc
1 glassful or 1 tumblerful	8 ounces	240 cc

NOTE: In solving problems where drams, ounces, and cc are involved, you must use equivalents from the table:

1 ounce = 8 drams = 30 or 32 cc

You may use 4 or 5 cc = 1 dram, but never 40 cc = 1 ounce.

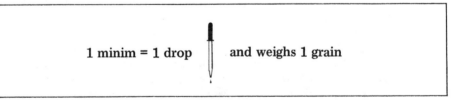

1 minim = 1 drop and weighs 1 grain

Figure 1. Equivalent units in the Apothecaries' System.

---

*Although most tables list 4 cc = 1 dram = 1 t and 4 t = 1 T, hospitals use medicine glasses and cups that are marked, "1 t = 5 cc, and 1 T = 15 cc"; hence, the two equivalents listed in the Metric system column and the occasional listing of 3 t = 1 T.

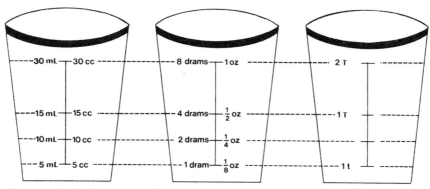

Figure 2. Equivalent quantities among the three systems of measurement shown in the form of 1-fluid-ounce medicine cups.

PRACTICE PROBLEMS

Supply the equivalents for the following

1. 2.2 lb = _____ kg   2. ℥ iv = _____ mL

3. 7½ lb = _____ g = _____ kg

4. 8 oz = _____ glassful

5. 1 T = _____ t = _____ drams

6. 1 oz = _____ mL = _____ drams

Convert the following:

7. 0.1 g = _____ mg   8. 0.25 liter = _____ mL

9. 100 mL = _____ liter   10. 100 mg = _____ g

Convert the following amounts:

11. ℥ ivss = _____ dram   12. grain iii = ℥ _____

13. m 180 = ℥ _____   14. ¼ pt = ℥ _____

Convert the following:

15. 0.016 g = _____ mg = _____ grain

16. grain $\dfrac{1}{300}$ = _____ mg = _____ g

17. grain x = _____ g = _____ mg

18. 20 mg = _____ g = _____ grain

19. 0.006 g = _____ grain = _____ mg

20. If 1 oz of solution contains grain xxx of a drug, how many grains does each dram contain? How many grams?

21. 1 t = _____ dram = _____ cc = _____ oz

22. 1 T = _____ oz = _____ dram = _____ cc

23. 1 glassful = _____ mL = _____ oz

Answers to Practice Problems

1. 1 kg

2. 16 mL

3. 3400 g or 3.4 kg (2.2 lb = 1 kg; so 7.5 ÷ 2.2 = 3.4 kg. Then move the decimal point three places to right, since 1000 g = 1 kg.)

4. 1 glassful

5. 4 t, 4 drams

6. 30–32 mL, 8 drams

7. 100 mg

8. 250 mL

9. 0.1 liter

10. 0.1 g

11. 36

12. ʒ $\frac{1}{20}$

13. ʒ iii

14. ʒ xxx

15. 16 mg, grain $\frac{1}{4}$

16. 0.2 mg, 0.0002 g

17. 0.6 g, 600 mg

18. 0.02 g, grain $\frac{1}{3}$

19. grain $\frac{1}{10}$, 6 mg

20. grain iv, 0.25 g

21. ʒ i, 4 cc, $\frac{1}{8}$ oz

22. ℥ ss, ʒ iv, 16 cc

23. 240 mL, 8 oz

If you made no more than four errors, go on to Lesson 5. If not, before proceeding do the Additional Practice Problems with no more than four errors.

ADDITIONAL PRACTICE PROBLEMS

Calculate the following:

1. Ounces in 1 glassful. _____

2. Milliliters in 1 glassful. _____

3. Cubic centimeters in ʒ ii. _____

4. Pounds in 40 kg. _____

Give the equivalents for the following amounts:

5. 320 mg = _____ g   6. 0.001 g = _____ mg

7. 16 mg = _____ g   8. 1 liter = _____ mL

9. 10 mL = _____ cc

Supply the equivalents in the Apothecaries' system for the following amounts:

10. ʒ ii = grain _____   11. *m* xxx = ʒ _____

12. 1 qt = _____ pt   13. 1 pt = _____ oz

Convert the amounts shown below:

14. grain i = _____ mg = _____ g

15. 0.5 g = _____ mg = _____ grain

16. ʒ ii = _____ cc = _____ drams

17. 0.5 liter = _____ mL = _____ pt

18. ʒ iv = _____ cc = _____ minims

19. If each dram of solution contains grain $\frac{1}{4}$ of a drug, how many milligrams per 4 cc? _____ How many g? _____

Give the equivalents for the following amounts:

20. 240 cc = _____ oz = _____ drams = _____ pt

21. 4–5 cc = _____ dram = _____ tsp

22. 1 oz = _____ tumblerful = _____ dram

23. 30 cc = _____ dram = _____ oz

24. If each ounce of solution contains 1 g of drug, how many milligrams are there in each dram? How many grains per dram?

Answers to Additional Practice Problems

1. 8 oz
2. 240 mL
3. 8 cc
4. 88 lb

5. 0.32 g
6. 1 mg
7. 0.016 g
8. 1000 mL
9. 10 cc

10. grain 120 or grain cxx
11. ℥ ss (or dr $\frac{1}{2}$)
12. 2 pt
13. 16 oz (or ℥ xvi)
14. 60 mg, 0.06 g
15. 500 mg, grain viiss (or grain $7\frac{1}{2}$)
16. 60 or 64 cc, 16 drams
    (or ℥ xvi)
17. 500 mL, 1 pt
18. 16 cc, 240 minims
19. 16 mg, 0.016 g
20. 8 oz, 64 drams, $\frac{1}{2}$ pt
21. 1 dram, 1 tsp
22. $\frac{1}{8}$ tumblerful, 8 drams
23. 8 drams, 1 oz

24. 125 mg per dram, grain ii per dram

LESSON 5

Review of Basic Arithmetic, Weights, and Measures

Objectives

By completing this review, the student will be able to:

- Demonstrate an understanding of basic arithmetic, weights, and measures, and Metric – Apothecaries' equivalents by solving the review problems with no more than seven errors. These problems should be solved without looking at a book.

REVIEW PROBLEMS

Which fraction is larger in value?

1. $\frac{1}{4}$ or $\frac{1}{6}$

2. $\frac{1}{100}$ or $\frac{1}{200}$

3. $\frac{3}{8}$ or $\frac{3}{4}$

4. $\frac{1}{60}$ or $\frac{1}{25}$

Circle the larger decimal fraction:

5. 0.425 or 0.4

6. 0.01 or 0.016

7. 0.05 or 0.005

8. 0.35 or 0.3

Write the following numbers as Roman numerals:

9. 64   10. 47   11. 38

Give Arabic numbers for each of the following:

12. LXXVIII   13. XIX   14. MCMLXXIX

15. If one tablet is grain $\frac{1}{4}$, how many grains in two tablets?

16. If one tablet is grain $\frac{1}{150}$, how many grains in one-half tablet?

17. How many sixths equal $\frac{1}{2}$?

18. If a solution has 0.60 g of drug in each dram, how many drams would you give for a dose of grain xxx?

Give the following equivalents in the Metric and Apothecaries' systems:

19. 0.1 g = _____mg = _____grains

20. grain xv = _____g = _____mg

21. 300 mg = _____g = _____grains

22. grain viiss = _____g = _____mg

23. 4 g = _____ mg = _____ grains

24. 1 oz = _____ mL = _____ minims = _____ drams

25. 1 tumblerful (glassful) = ___240___ mL

Change the following to decimal fractions, percents, fractions, and ratios:

Percent	Decimal Fraction	Fraction	Ratio
26. _____	27. _____	28. $\frac{1}{2}$	29. _____
30. _____	31. 0.05	32. _____	33. _____
34. _____	35. _____	36. _____	37. 1 : 4
38. $\frac{1}{2}\%$	39. _____	40. _____	41. _____

42. How many cubic centimeters in 0.5 liter?

43. 0.008 g is what part of 0.016 g?

44. If a newborn infant weighs 4500 g, what is the weight in pounds and ounces? (16 oz = 1 lb)

45. The physician orders 0.5 g of sulfadiazine to be taken by mouth. The tablets available are grain viiss, 500 mg, and 1 g each. Which tablet would you choose and how many would you give?

46. Common units of the Metric system are _____, _____, _____, and _____.

Give equivalents for the following:

47. 1 qt = _____ pt = _____ gal = _____ mL

48. 1 pt = _____ cc = _____ qt = _____ gal

49. 0.008 g = _____ mg = _____ grains

50. If a patient is taking 100 mg of a drug every 3 hours, how many *grains* will he take in 24 hours? How many grams?

Solve the following problems:

51. $x : 5 :: 4 : 2$ 52. $0.2 : 5000 :: 2 : x$

53. If the physician orders fluids increased to 3000 cc per 24 hours, how many tumblersful (glassfuls) should the patient receive in 24 hours?

Answers to Review Problems

1. $\dfrac{1}{4}$ 2. $\dfrac{1}{100}$

3. $\dfrac{3}{4}$ 4. $\dfrac{1}{25}$

5. 0.425   6. 0.016

7. 0.05   8. 0.35

9. LXIV   10. XLVII   11. XXXVIII

12. 78   13. 19   14. 1979

15. grain $\dfrac{1}{2}$

16. grain $\dfrac{1}{300}$ [Did you miss this one? Remember, $\dfrac{1}{2} \times \dfrac{1}{150} = \dfrac{1}{300}$.

Multiply numerators together and then denominators.]

17. $\dfrac{3}{6} = \dfrac{1}{2}$ [Easy, wasn't it?]

18. 3 drams [0.65 g = grain x = 1 dram. So, grain xxx = 3 drams.]

19. 100 mg, grain iss ($1\frac{1}{2}$)   20. 1 g, 1000 mg
21. 0.3 g, grain v   22. 0.5 g, 500 mg
23. 4000 mg, grain lx   24. 30 mL, 480 minims, 8 drams
25. 240 mL

26. 50%   27. 0.5   28. $\dfrac{1}{2}$ 29. $1 : 2$

30. 5%   31. 0.05   32. $\dfrac{1}{20}$ 33. $1 : 20$

34. 25%   35. 0.25   36. $\dfrac{1}{4}$ 37. $1 : 4$

38. $\dfrac{1}{2}\%$ 39. 0.005   40. $\dfrac{1}{200}$

41. 1 : 200
42. 500 cc

43. $\dfrac{1}{2}$ (0.008 + 0.008 = 0.016)

44. 4500 g = 4.5 kg × 2.2 lb = 9.9 lb or 9 lb, 14 oz
45. grain viiss or 500 mg. Give one of either.
46. mg, g, mL, cc

47. 2 pt, $\dfrac{1}{4}$ gal, 1000 mL

48. 500 cc, $\dfrac{1}{2}$ qt, $\dfrac{1}{8}$ gal

49. 8 mg, grain $\dfrac{1}{8}$

50. q 3 hr × 24 hr = 8 doses × 100 mg per dose = 800 mg ÷ 60 = 13.3 grains or 0.8 g

51. $x = 10$ 52. $x = 50,000$
53. $12\frac{1}{2}$ tumblersful

If you made no more than seven errors, go on to Lesson 6. If not, do the Additional Review Problems with no more than six errors before proceeding.

ADDITIONAL REVIEW PROBLEMS

Which fraction is larger:

1. $\dfrac{2}{3}$ or $\dfrac{3}{4}$ 2. $\dfrac{1}{100}$ or $\dfrac{1}{150}$

3. $\dfrac{7}{8}$ or $\dfrac{5}{6}$ 4. $\dfrac{3}{8}$ or $\dfrac{1}{4}$

Circle the larger decimal fraction:

5. 0.325 or 0.2   6. 0.02 or 0.025   7. 0.008 or 0.006

Write the following numbers as Roman numerals:

8. 59 _____   9. 88 _____   10. 4 _____

Write the following as Arabic numerals:

11. XLIV _____   12. XXIX _____   13. XC _____

14. If one tablet is grain $\frac{1}{150}$, what do two tablets equal?

15. How many eighths equal $\frac{3}{6}$?

16. If a bottle of medicine has grain $\frac{1}{4}$ in each dram, how many drams would you give for a dosage of grain $\frac{3}{4}$?

Give the following equivalents in the Metric and Apothecaries' systems:

17. grain $\dfrac{1}{100}$ = _____ mg = _____ g

18. 1 cc = _____ mL = _____ minims

19. 1 glassful = _____ cc = _____ dram = _____ oz

20. 0.05 g = _____ mg = _____ grains

21. Change 1 qt, 1 pt to the Metric system.

22. If one tablet is 0.5 g, how many grams in two tablets?

23. In a solution labeled grain x per dram, how much would be needed to give grain v? grain xv?

24. If 1 oz of solution contains 60 grains of drug, how much is in each dram?

25. If a newborn infant weighs 2500 g, what is the baby's weight in pounds and ounces?

26. The physician orders elixir of terpin hydrate with codeine grain ss. The bottle on hand is labeled 60 mg codeine per dram. How many drams would you give?

27. If the physician orders dihydromorphine (Dilaudid) grain $\frac{1}{32}$, would you give 2 tablets grain $\frac{1}{16}$ each or 2 tablets grain $\frac{1}{64}$ each?

Give the following equivalents in the Metric and Apothecaries' systems:

28. grain xxx = _____ mg = _____ g

29. grain v = _____ mg = _____ g

30. 0.5 cc = _____ minims

31. 1 tumblerful = _____ mL = _____ oz

Solve the following problems:

32. $0.05 : 1000 :: 1 : x$ 33. $\dfrac{1}{100} : 2 :: \dfrac{1}{150} : x$

Change the following to alternate forms:

Percent	Decimal Fraction	Fraction	Ratio
34. _____	35. _____	36. $\dfrac{1}{20}$	37. _____
38. _____	39. 0.005	40. _____	41. _____
42. 25%	43. _____	44. _____	45. _____
46. _____	47. _____	48. _____	49. 1 : 200

50. Elixir of phenobarbital has 16 mg per dram. The physician orders 4 cc every 4 hours. How many milligrams does the patient receive per dose? How many grains?

51. The physician has ordered aspirin 0.6 g, and the tablets are labeled "300 mg each." How many would you give?

Answers to Additional Review Problems

1. $\dfrac{3}{4}$ 2. $\dfrac{1}{100}$

3. $\dfrac{7}{8}$ 4. $\dfrac{3}{8}$

5. 0.325   6. 0.025   7. 0.008
8. LIX   9. LXXXVIII   10. IV
11. 44   12. 29   13. 90

14. grain $\frac{1}{75}$ [You didn't miss this one? Remember, when adding fractions, add the numerators, leave the denominators the same, and reduce to lowest terms.]

15. $\frac{4}{8} = \frac{3}{6} = \frac{1}{2}$

16. ʒiii (or 3 drams) [ʒi = grain $\frac{1}{4}$. Therefore, ʒiii = grain $\frac{3}{4}$.]

17. 0.6 mg, 0.0006 g   18. 1 mL, 15 or 16 minims
19. 240 cc, 60 drams, 8 oz   20. 50 mg, $\frac{5}{6}$ grain

21. 1 qt = 1000 cc
    1 pt = $\underline{500\text{ cc}}$
             1500 cc

22. 1 g

23. ʒ ss, ʒ iss

24. grain viiss [Remember, 1 oz = 8 drams. Then, 60 ÷ 8 = $7\frac{1}{2}$ grains.]

25. $5\frac{1}{2}$ lb

26. ʒ ss

27. 2 tablets grain $\frac{1}{64}$ each [If you chose 2 tablets grain $\frac{1}{16}$ each: $\frac{1}{16} + \frac{1}{16} = \frac{2}{16} = \frac{1}{8}$, or 4 times the dose ordered.]

28. 1800 mg, 1.8 g   29. 300 mg, 0.3 g
30. 8 minims   31. 240 mL, 8 oz
32. $x = 20{,}000$ 33. $x = 1\frac{1}{3}$

34. 5%   35. 0.05   36. $\dfrac{1}{20}$ 37. 1 : 20

38. 0.5%   39. 0.005   40. $\dfrac{1}{200}$ 41. 1 : 200

42. 25%   43. 0.25   44. $\dfrac{1}{4}$ 45. 1 : 4

46. $\frac{1}{2}$%   47. 0.005   48. $\dfrac{1}{200}$ 49. 1 : 200

50. ʒi = 16 mg [ʒi = 4 cc. So, the patient receives 16 mg or grain $\frac{1}{4}$.]

51. 2 tablets, 300 mg [0.6 g = 600 mg]

LESSON 6

Computing the Dosage of Oral Medications

Objectives

After completing this lesson, and without referring to a book, the student will be able to:

- Write the formula for determining the number of tablets or capsules to be given.

- Compute the total number of tablets or capsules to order for the number of days prescribed.

- Compute dosage for drugs to be given orally.

- Compute the amount of liquid to be given when the order is written in grains, milligrams, or grams.

- Solve the practice problems at the end of this lesson with no more than two errors.

The most common method for the administration of drugs is by mouth. Preparations of drugs for oral administration may be in solid form, such as pills, tablets, or capsules, or in liquid form. Sometimes the nurse must compute the dosage for drugs given orally because the amount of the drug available is expressed in a different measure than that ordered. The available drug may be smaller than that ordered or the drug may be in solution and expressed only as a percent.

TABLETS AND CAPSULES

The physician may write the number of grains, grams, or milligrams to be given and not state the number of tablets or capsules. Therefore, the nurse must determine how many tablets or capsules to give the patient, and may also have to determine the total number of tablets or capsules to order for the number of days the medication is prescribed.

EXAMPLE: Physician's order, "Sulfadiazine 4 g initially, then 0.5 g q 6 hr × 3 days." Determine how many tablets to order.

Sulfadiazine is available in 300- and 500-mg tablets. Since the 0.5 g is ordered every 6 hours and 500 mg = 0.5 g, the 500-mg tablet is the dosage of choice. Next, the nurse must determine how many tablets are needed for the 3-day supply. Since the initial dose is 4 g and each tablet is 0.5 g: 4.0 ÷ 0.5 = 8 tablets initially. Then, since q 6 hr means 4 times a day:

1 tablet × 4 times a day × 3 days = 12 tablets

Thus, 8 tablets initially plus 12 tablets subsequently equals a total of 20 tablets to order.

To determine the number of capsules or tablets to administer, use the following proportion formula:

$$\frac{\text{Dose Ordered}}{\text{Dose on Hand}} :: \frac{\text{Capsules per Dose}}{\text{Drug Form (cap, tab)}} = \frac{\text{Number of Tablets}}{\text{or Capsules per Dose}}$$

or, the proportion formula shortened:

$$\frac{\text{Dose Ordered}}{\text{Dose on Hand}} \times \text{Drug form (cap, tab)} = \frac{\text{Number of Tablets}}{\text{or Capsules per Dose}}$$

EXAMPLE: Physician's order, "Aspirin grain x q 4 hr." The aspirin is labeled, "0.3 g per tablet."

First convert grains to grams, or grams to grains (16 grains = 1 g):

10 grains = 10 ÷ 16 = 0.6 g

The solution is then

$$\frac{\text{Dose Ordered}}{\text{Dose on Hand}} \times 1 \text{ tablet} = \frac{0.6 \text{ g}}{0.3 \text{ g}} \times 1 = 2 \text{ tablets}$$

NOTE: Fractions of capsules are not given, since a capsule cannot be divided accurately into halves, thirds, fourths, etc. If your answer is $3\frac{1}{4}$, for example, you would give 3 capsules, or if 3.7, you would give 4 capsules. Occasionally, one-half of a tablet may be given, since some tablets are scored to allow easy division in half, but smaller units cannot be divided accurately.

LIQUIDS

EXAMPLE: Physician's order, "Elixir phenobarbital grain ss q 4 hr." The drug available, or stock solution, is labeled, "Elixir of phenobarbital 16 mg per 4 cc."

In this problem there are two steps; the grains must be converted to milligrams or the milligrams to grains:

60 or 64 mg = 1 grain

32 mg = grain $\overline{\text{ss}}$

If 16 mg = 4 cc, then 32 mg or grain ss = 8 cc. This problem can be solved without using a formula.

Or substituting the values given into the formula presented above, you would have the following:

$$\frac{\text{Dose Ordered}}{\text{Dose on Hand}} \times \text{Drug Form} = \frac{\overset{2}{\cancel{32}} \text{ mg}}{\cancel{16} \text{ mg}} \times 4 \text{ cc} = 8 \text{ cc}$$

EXAMPLE: Physician's order, "Elixir terpin hydrate with codeine grain ss q 4 hr." The bottle is labeled, "Elixir terpin hydrate with codeine 16 mg per dram."

Remembering that $\frac{1}{2}$ grain = 32 mg and substituting in the formula, you would have the following:

$$\frac{\text{Dose Ordered}}{\text{Dose on Hand}} \times \text{Drug Form (dram)} = \frac{\overset{2}{\cancel{32}} \text{ mg}}{\cancel{16} \text{ mg}} \times 1 \text{ dram} = 2 \text{ drams}$$

The patient would thus receive 2-dram doses.

EXAMPLE: Physician's order, "Chloral hydrate syrup grain viiss tid." The label on bottle reads, "Chloral hydrate syrup 10% solution."

There are several steps in this problem. First, you have to determine the amount of drug in a 10% solution. A 10% solution means there are 10 parts of drug to 100 parts of water, that is, a proportion of 10 : 100 or, reduced to its smallest form, 1 : 10. Since the dose ordered is grain viiss, which equals 0.5 g, 1 g per 10 cc would be more convenient values with which to work. Substituting the quantities from the problem into the formula:

$$\frac{\text{Dose Ordered}}{\text{Dose on Hand}} \times \text{Drug Form} = \frac{0.5\text{ g}}{1\text{ g}} \times 10\text{ cc} = 5\text{ cc}$$

(The quantity of 10 cc is the amount of solution in which drug is dissolved—a 10% solution.)

NOTE: Proportions can be set up only when equivalent amounts in the same system are used—grains and minims, or grams and cubic centimeters. That is, all the units must belong to either the Metric or the Apothecaries' system, and they must also be equivalent in that system.

Before you continue with dosage problems, you will need to *memorize* the following Metric–Apothecaries' equivalents:

---

1 g = 1000 mg = 15 or 16 grains
60 or 64 mg = 1 grain
1 mL or cc = 15 or 16 minims

Since 1 minim weighs approximately 1 grain and 1 cc or mL weighs approximately 1 g, then 1 cc and 1 g, and 1 minim and 1 grain are essentially equivalent, but are not equal as one is solid measure and one is liquid measure.

---

1 dram = 4 or 5 cc
8 drams = 1 oz = 30 or 32 cc
1 teaspoonful = 1 dram = 4 or 5 cc
1 tablespoonful = 3 or 4 drams = 15 or 16 cc

PRACTICE PROBLEMS

Tablets and Capsules

1. The physician orders 1.5 mg tablets to be taken by mouth. The tablets available are 0.5 and 0.75 mg. Which would you give and how many? Justify your answer.

2. The physician's order is, "Methacycline (Rondomycin) 0.3 g initially, then 150 mg q 6 hr × 3 days." Methacycline is available in 150- and 300-mg capsules. Determine the number of capsules per dose and the total number to order for the 3-day supply.

3. The physician orders "Aspirin (acetylsalicylic acid) grain X qid (4 times a day) for 7 days." The pharmacy has 300- and 600-mg tablets. Which tablet would you give and how many would you order for the 7-day supply?

4. The physician's order is, "Chloramphenicol capsules (Chloromycetin) 0.5 g q 6 hr × 3 days." Chloramphenicol is available in 50-, 100-, and 250-mg capsules. Determine which of the capsules to order, the total number to order, and how many to administer for each dose.

5. If a patient receives a total of 4 g of sulfathiazole (Sulfamul) in 24 hours, how many *grains* does he receive? If the medication is given every 6 hours, how many grains does the patient receive each dose? How many grams?

Liquids

6. The physician's order is, "Elixir phenobarbital grain i q 4 hr." The bottle is labeled, "Elixir phenobarbital 32 mg per dram." How many drams would you give per dose?

7. The physician's order is, "Elixir ferrous sulfate 600 mg tid (3 times a day) with meals. Have patient drink through a straw." The label on the bottle is, "Elixir ferrous sulfate, 300 mg per 10 mL." How many milliliters would the patient receive per dose? How many drams per dose?

8. The physician's order is, "Potassium triplex 30 mEq in glass fruit juice tid (3 times a day)." The label reads, "15 mEq per 5 mL." How many milliliters would you administer for each dose?

9. The physician's order is, "Elixir sodium bromide 300 mg tid, pc (3 times a day after meals)." The label reads: "700 mg per 4 mL." How many milliliters of sodium bromide would the patient receive each dose?

10. The physician orders potassium gluconate elixir 40 mEq qid (4 times a day). The bottle is labeled, "Potassium gluconate 20 mEq per 15 mL." How many milliliters would you give per dose? How many *drams* per dose?

11. The physician orders, "Chloral hydrate syrup grain viiss, tid ($7\frac{1}{2}$ grains, 3 times a day)." The label reads, "Chloral hydrate syrup 500 mg per dram." How many *drams* would you give per dose? If you were instructing a member of the family to administer this when the patient goes home, how many *teaspoonsful* should the patient receive for a dose of 500 mg?

Answers to Practice Problems

1. 0.75 mg, 2 tablets. [You would need 3 tablets of 0.5 mg.]
2. Use the 150-mg tablets: 2 tablets per dose, 14 tablets for a 3-day supply. [Although 0.3 g = 300 mg, the subsequent doses are 150 mg, and it is thus more convenient to use the smaller quantity. Then,

$$300 \div 150 = 2$$

$$72 \div 6 = 12 \times 1 = 12$$

Thus, 2 tablets + 12 tablets = 14 tablets.]
3. 600-mg tablet, 28 tablets for 7-day supply. [If 1 grain = 60 mg, then 10 ∧ grains = 600 mg. Thus, 1 tablet × 4 times a day × 7 days = 28 capsules.]
4. Order 24 of the 250-mg capsules; give 2 capsules per dose. [First, 0.5 g = 500 mg. Then,

$$500 \div 250 = 2.$$

Finally,

2 capsules × 4 times a day (q 6 hr) × 3 days = 24 capsules.]

5. 60 grains total. 15 grains per dose, 1 g per dose. [4 g × 15 = 60 grains. Add 24 ÷ 6 = 4 doses; then 60 ÷ 4 = 15 grains = 1 g.]
6. ʒ ii. [ʒ i = 32 mg = grain ½; 64 mg = grain i = ʒ ii]
7. 20 mL or ʒ v
8. 10 mL
9. 1.7 mL
10. 30 mL or 8 drams
11. ʒ i (ʒ i = 1 t = 500 mg)

If you made no more than two errors, go on to Lesson 7. If not, do the Additional Practice Problems with no more than two errors before proceeding.

ADDITIONAL PRACTICE PROBLEMS

Tablets and Capsules

1. Physician's order, "Tetracycline 0.3 g q 12 hr for 4 days. Give po with full glass of water 2 hours pc (after meals)." The medication is labeled, "Demeclocyline (tetracycline) 150-mg capsules." State the number of capsules per dose and the number to order for the 4-day supply.

2. Physician's order, "Sodium dicloxacillin monohydrate (Veracillin) 0.25 g q 6 hr with full glass water 2 hours pc" Drug available as 250-mg cap. How many capsules will you give for each dose?

3. Physician's order: "Erythromycin 500 mg q 6 hr for 4 days." Drug available as 250-mg tab. State the number of tablets per dose and the number to order for the 4-day supply.

4. Physician's order, "Guanethidine (Ismelin) 0.025 g od (once a day)." Drug available as 25-mg tab. State how many tablets you would give each dose.

5. Physician's order, "Kanamycin grain xv q 6 hr for 3 days." Drug available as kanamycin sulfate 500-mg cap. How many would you give for each dose and how many would you order for the 3-day supply?

6. Physician's order: "Liotrix (levothyroxine 0.0125 mg and liothyronine 0.0031 mg) once daily." Drug available as levothyroxine 12.5 μg plus liothyronine 3.1 μg (Note: Liotrix is a tablet which contains both medications.) How many tablets would you give daily?

7. Physician's order: "Methocarbamol 1.5 g od" Drug available as 750-mg tablets. How many would you give per dose and how many would you order for a 7-day supply?

Liquids

8. Physician's order, "Erythromycin oral suspension 0.4 g q 6 hr." Drug available is ethylsuccinate oral suspension (erythromycin) 400 mg per 5 mL. How many milliliters would the patient receive per dose? How many milligrams would the patient receive in 24 hours?

9. Physician's order, "Hydroxyzine syrup 75 mg q 4 hr." Drug available is hydroxyzine hydrochloride syrup 10 mg per 5 mL. How many drams would you give per dose? How many milliliters?

10. Physician's order, "Isoniazid syrup 0.3 g od" Drug is available as isoniazid syrup 50 mg per 5 mL. How many milliliters per dose? How many milligrams per dose? How many drams per dose?

11. Physician's order, "Theophylline elixir 100 mg bid (twice daily)." Drug is available as theophylline elixir 0.05 g per 5 mL. How many milliliters would you give per dose? How many grams per dose?

12. Physician's order, "Potassium gluconate elixir 20 mEq qid" Drug is available as potassium gluconate elixir 20 mEq per 15 mL. How many milliliters would the patient receive daily?

13. Physician's order, "Pentobarbital elixir 0.1 g hs (at bedtime). Drug is available as pentobarbital elixir 20 mg per 5 mL. How many milliliters would you give each dose?

Answers to Additional Practice Problems

1. 2 cap, 150 mg each, per dose; 16 cap to order for 4 days
2. 1 cap, 250 mg per dose
3. 2 tab, 250 mg each, per dose; 32 tablets for 4-day supply
4. 1 tab, 25 mg per dose
5. 2 cap, 500 mg each, per dose; 24 cap for 3-day supply
6. 1 tab, daily
7. 2 tab, 750 mg each, per dose; 14 tab for 7-day supply

8. 5 mL per dose. [400 mg q 6 hr × 4 doses = 1600 mg/24 hr.]
9. ℥ viiss per dose, 37.5 mL per dose. [Remember, 4–5 mL = ℥ i.]
10. 30 mL per dose, 300 mg per dose, 8 drams per dose
11. 10 mL per dose, 0.1 g per dose
12. 60 mL per day. [15 mL × 4 times a day = 60 mL]
13. 100 mg per dose, 25 mL per dose

LESSON 7

Computing Dosages of Parenteral Medications

Objectives

After completing this lesson, and without referring to a book, the student will be able to:

- Compute dosage for injection from prepared solutions.

- Solve the practice problems at the end of this lesson with no more than three errors.

Parenteral medications are drugs that are given by injection. The usual routes of administration are intramuscular, subcutaneous, or intravenous. Preparations of drugs for injection come in ampules or single- or multiple-dose vials with the drug either in solution, powder, or crystals. The amount of drug dissolved may be given in grains, milligrams, grams, units, or milliequivalents. The amounts of solution are not standardized and may range from less than 0.5 cc to 50 cc.

There are two formulas which may be used in the calculation of dosage from prepared solutions. You may use whichever seems easier for you.

Formula 1

Drug on Hand : Dilution :: Drug Ordered : x

NOTE: Dilution is the amount of solution in which the (unit of) drug is dissolved.

Formula 2

$$\frac{\text{Dose Ordered}}{\text{Drug on Hand}} \times \text{Dilution or Amount of Solution}$$

Formula 2 is a shortened form of the method of Formula 1, eliminating steps 1 and 2 in the proportion formula. Formula 2 is actually step 3 of the proportion formula. Some examples using these two formulas are given below.

EXAMPLE: The physician orders morphine 10 mg. The drug available is morphine 16 mg per 1-cc ampule.

Using dosage Formula 1, substitute the values given:

16 mg : 1 cc :: 10 mg : x

Then multiply the extremes and means and solve the resulting equation for x:

$16x = 10$

$x = 0.6$ cc (or m x)

$$0.6 \text{ cc} \times 16 \; m = \frac{6}{\overset{}{\underset{5}{10}}} \times \overset{8}{16} = \frac{48}{5} = 9.6 \text{ or } m \text{ x}$$

Thus, you should draw up and administer 10 minims, which contains 10 mg morphine; you would then discard the remaining 6 minims in the ampule.

If the amount of solution in which the drug is dissolved is not 1 cc or 1 mL, that amount should be substituted in the formula.

EXAMPLE: The physician's order is, "Meperidine (Demerol) 75 mg IM now." Ampule is labeled, "Meperidine hydrochloride 100 mg per 2 mL."

You can substitute the values given in Formula 1 and solve the resulting equation as follows:

$$100 \text{ mg} : 2 \text{ cc} :: 75 \text{ mg} : x$$

$$100x = 150$$

$$x = 1.5 \text{ cc}$$

Or you can use Formula 2.

$$\frac{\text{Dose Ordered}}{\text{Dose on Hand}} \times \text{Dilution} = \frac{\overset{3}{\cancel{75}} \text{ mg}}{\underset{4}{\cancel{100}} \text{ mg}} \times 2 \text{ cc} = \frac{6}{4} = 1.5 \text{ cc}$$

Answer: Draw up 1.5 cc of solution, which contains 75 mg of drug, and discard the remaining 0.5 cc.

EXAMPLE: The physician's order is, "Caffeine sodium benzoate grain v stat." The label on the ampule is, "Caffeine sodium benzoate 0.5 g per 5 cc."

First, grain v must be converted to grams:

$$5 \text{ grains} \div 15 \text{ grains} = 0.3 \text{ g}$$

Now with all the units in one system, you can substitute the values into Formula 2:

$$\frac{0.3 \text{ g}}{0.5 \text{ g}} \times 5 \text{ cc} = 3 \text{ cc}$$

NOTE: When stock solutions are used, usually in vials of 5 or 10 mL, you calculate the dosage needed and withdraw that amount from the vial.

EXAMPLE: The physician orders 2 g of a medication, and the drug is available as a 20% solution.

A 20% solution means there are 20 g drug per 100 mL of solution (20 : 100), which reduces to 1 g per 5 mL. If 1 g = 5 mL, then 2 g = 10 mL. Alternatively,

$$\frac{20}{100} \div 10 = 2 \text{ per 10 mL}$$

EXAMPLE: Give ephedrine sulfate grain $\frac{3}{4}$ and the drug available is ephedrine sulfate grain $\frac{3}{8}$ per 1 mL ampule.

Now it is obvious that you cannot get $\frac{3}{4}$ out of $\frac{3}{8}$, so two ampules are needed. Two ampules of ephedrine sulfate grain $\frac{3}{8}$ each will equal grain $\frac{3}{4}$, so no calculation is necessary ($\frac{3}{8} + \frac{3}{8} = \frac{6}{8} = \frac{3}{4}$). Or, substituting in Formula 2:

$$\frac{\text{Drug Ordered}\left(\text{grain } \dfrac{3}{4}\right)}{\text{Drug on Hand}\left(\text{grain } \dfrac{3}{8}\right)} \times \text{Amount Solution (1 cc)} =$$

$$\frac{3}{\cancel{4}} \times \frac{\overset{2}{\cancel{8}}}{\cancel{3}} \times 1 \text{ cc} = 2 \text{ cc}$$

As we already know, 2 cc (two ampules) contain grain $\frac{3}{4}$.

EXAMPLE: Give 400,000 units of penicillin G from a 5-mL vial containing 1,000,000 units.

Substituting in the formula:

$$\frac{\overset{2}{\cancel{400,000}} \text{ units}}{\underset{5}{\cancel{1,000,000}} \text{ units}} \times \cancel{5} \text{ mL} = 2 \text{ mL}$$

Answer: Draw up 2 mL of penicillin G, which contains 400,000 units, and administer to patient.

NOTE: Dilution may range from 0.5 to 20 mL, so read problem carefully for the amount of solution in which medication is dissolved.

EXAMPLE: The physician's preoperative order is, "Atropine sulfate grain $\frac{1}{150}$ and meperidine hydrochloride (Demerol) 50 mg IM @ 7:30 AM." The drugs available are atropine sulfate 0.6 mg per cc and meperidine 100 mg per 2 cc.

This example is worked as two separate problems, but the drugs are administered in the same syringe. Calculating first for atropine, the problem can be worked by changing grain $\frac{1}{150}$ to milligrams:

$$\text{grain } \frac{1}{\underset{5}{\cancel{150}}} \times \overset{2}{\cancel{60}} \text{ mg} = \frac{2}{5} = 0.4 \text{ mg}$$

Then substituting in the formula:

$$\frac{\text{Drug Ordered}}{\text{Drug on Hand}} \times \text{Dilution} = \frac{0.4 \text{ mg}}{0.6 \text{ mg}} \times 1 \text{ cc} = \frac{\overset{2}{\cancel{4}}}{\underset{3}{\cancel{6}}} \times 1 \text{ cc}$$

$$= \frac{2}{3} \text{ cc or 10 minims, which contains 0.4 mg or}$$

$$\text{grain } \frac{1}{150} \text{ of atropine}$$

Or you can change the 0.6 mg of available drug to grains and then substitute in the formula:

$$\frac{0.6 \text{ mg}}{60 \text{ mg}} = \frac{\cancel{6}}{10} \times \frac{1}{\underset{10}{\cancel{60}}} = \frac{1}{100} \text{ grain}$$

$$\frac{\text{grain } \frac{1}{150}}{\text{grain } \frac{1}{100}} \times 1 \text{ cc} = \text{grain } \frac{1}{\underset{3}{\cancel{150}}} \times \text{grain } \frac{\overset{2}{\cancel{100}}}{1} \times 1 \text{ cc} = \frac{2}{3} \text{ cc or } m \text{ x}$$

(Invert divisor before multiplying.)

Draw up 10 minims atropine sulfate from the ampule which contains 0.6 mg atropine per cc. The 10 minims of solution will contain 0.4 mg. Next, the meperidine dosage required can be done mentally (if 2 cc = 100 mg, then 1 cc = 50 mg), or the problem can be worked by formula:

$$\frac{\text{Dose Ordered}}{\text{Drug on Hand}} \times \text{Dilution} = \frac{\cancel{50} \text{ mg}}{\underset{2}{\cancel{100}} \text{ mg}} \times \overset{1}{\cancel{2}} \text{ cc} = 1 \text{ cc}$$

NOTE: *The dilution here is 2 cc, since there are 100 mg per 2 cc.*

EXAMPLE: The physician orders 0.2 mg digoxin (H). The drug available is 0.5 mg per mL.

Substituting in the formula:

$$\frac{0.2 \text{ mg}}{0.5 \text{ mg}} \times 1 \text{ mL} = \frac{2}{5} \times 1 \text{ mL} = 0.4 \text{ mL or 6 minims}$$

Answer: Draw up 6 minims (*m* vi) of solution from the ampule labeled "Digoxin 0.5 mg per mL." The 6 minims will contain 0.2 mg digoxin.

EXAMPLE: The physician orders potassium chloride 12 mEq bid. The vial is labeled, "Potassium chloride 20 mEq per 10 mL."

Substituting in the formula:

$$\frac{\overset{6}{\cancel{12}} \text{ mEq}}{\underset{2}{\cancel{20}} \text{ mEq}} \times \cancel{10} \text{ mL} = 6 \text{ mL}$$

NOTE: The dilution in this problem is 10 mL.

Answer: Draw up 6 mL, which will contain 12 mEq potassium chloride.

PRACTICE PROBLEMS

Each of the following problems gives the physician's orders and the amounts in which the drugs are available. For each problem, calculate the correct dose and state your answer in the following form:
Draw up 0.5 mL (which equals 8 mg) from ampule which has grain $\frac{1}{4}$ per 1 mL.

1. "Compazine grain $\frac{1}{6}$ IM now." The ampule is labeled, "Prochlorperazine edisylate (Compazine) 5 mg per mL." How many milliliters would you give?

2. "Dilaudid grain $\frac{1}{32}$ q 4 hr prn for pain." The drug available is labeled "Hydromorphine hydrochloride (Dilaudid) 2 mg per mL." How many minims would you give?

3. "Gentamicin sulfate 80 mg IM q 12 hr." The gentamicin is available as 0.08 g per mL.

4. "Aminophylline 0.5 g IM q 4 hr prn for asthma." The drug available is labeled, "Aminophylline grain viiss per 2-cc ampule."

5. "Tigan 200 mg IM stat (at once)." Drug is labeled, "Trimethobenzamide hydrochloride (Tigan) 0.1 g per mL."

6. "Wycillin 500,000 units IM bid (twice a day)." Drug available is procaine penicillin G (Wycillin) in 10-cc vial with 300,000 units per mL.

7. "Cedilanid D 0.6 mg IM qd (once daily)." Drug available is deslanoside (Cedilanid) 0.8 mg per 4-mL ampule.

8. "Calcium gluconate 1 g IV stat." Drug available is calcium gluconate 10%, 10-mL vial.

9. "Levo-Dromoran 1.5 mg subcutaneously q 6 hr prn for pain." Drug available is levorphanol tartrate (Levo-Dromoran) 2 mg per mL.

10. Preoperative medication: Demerol 75 mg and atropine sulfate 0.4 mg on call to the Operating Room. Drugs available: meperidine hydrochloride (De-

merol) 100 mg per 2 mL and atropine sulfate grain $\frac{1}{150}$ per mL. (These are worked as two separate problems but are administered in the same syringe.)

11. "Quinidine grain ii stat." Drug available is quinidine gluconate 80 mg per mL.

12. "Valium 5 mg IM now." Drug available: diazepam (Valium) 0.01 g per mL.

13. "Regitine grain $\frac{1}{12}$ IM now." Drug available: phentolamine hydrochloride (Regitine) 5 mg per mL.

14. "Ephedrine sulfate grain $\frac{3}{8}$ IM stat." Drug available: ephedrine sulfate 50 mg per mL.

15. "Kantrex grain xv IM q 6 hr." Drug available: kanamycin sulfate (Kantrex) 0.5 g per 2 mL.

16. "Methergine 0.2 mg IM stat." Drug available: methylergonovine (methergine) grain $\frac{1}{320}$ per mL.

17. "Narcan 0.2 mg IM stat." Drug available: Narcan 0.4 mg per 1-mL ampule.

18. "Protamine sulfate 50 mg now." Drug available: protamine sulfate 0.05 g per mL.

19. "Declomycin 150 mg IM now and q 6 hr." Drug available: demeclocycline hydrochloride (Declomycin) 0.15 g per mL.

20. "Solu Cortef 200 mg IM q 6 hr." Drug available: hydrocortisone sodium succinate (Solu Cortef) 0.3 g per 2 mL.

21. "Parathyroid hormone 30 units IM q 12 hr." Drug available: parathyroid hormone 100 units per mL.

22. "Aramine 4 mg IM stat." Drug available: metaraminol bitartrate (Aramine) 0.01 g per mL.

23. "Atropine sulfate grain $\frac{1}{150}$ (H) stat." Drug available: atropine sulfate 0.6 mg per mL.

24. "Epinephrine hydrochloride 1 : 1000 IM stat." Drug available: epinephrine hydrochloride 0.1% solution in 1-mL ampule.

25. "Phenobarbital sodium grain iii @ 8 AM" Drug available: phenobarbital sodium 325 mg per mL.

Answers to Practice Problems

1. 2 mL (Draw up 2 mL, which equals grain $\frac{1}{6}$ or 10 mg.)
2. 1 mL or 16 minims (64 mg per grain was used in this problem because it cancels evenly.)
3. 1 mL 0.08 g = 80 mg (Draw up 1 mL = 80 mg.)
4. 2 cc grain viiss = 0.5 g (Draw up 2 cc = 0.5 g.)
5. 2 mL 0.1 g = 100 mg (Draw up 2 mL = 100 mg.)
6. 1.6 mL (Draw up 1.6 mL, which = 500,000 units.)
7. 3 mL (Draw up 3 mL which = 0.6 mg.)
8. 10 mL 10% solution = 10 : 100 or 1 g per 10 mL solution
9. 0.75 mL or 12 minims (m xii) (Draw up 0.75 mL or m xii = 1.5 mg.)
10. 1.5 mL meperidine and 1 mL atropine sulfate. (Draw up 1.5 mL of meperidine = 75 mg and 1 mL atropine = 0.4 mg.)
11. 1.5 mL (grain ii = 120 mg. Then, $\dfrac{120\ \text{mg}}{80} \times 1\ \text{mL} = 1.5\ \text{mL} = 80\ \text{mg}$.)
12. 0.5 mL (Draw up 0.5 mL = 5 mg.)
13. 1 mL grain $\frac{1}{12} \times 60\ \text{mg} = 5\ \text{mg}$ (Draw up 1 mL = 5 mg.)
14. 0.5 mL (Draw up 0.5 mL = grain $\frac{3}{8}$ [This is an example of the discrepancy in Metric–Apothecaries' equivalents.]

$$\text{grain } \frac{3}{\cancel{8}} \times \overset{8}{\cancel{64}}\ \text{mg} = 24\ \text{mg}$$

$$\frac{24\ \text{mg}}{50\ \text{mg}} \times 1\ \text{mL} = 0.48\ \text{mL} \text{ which should be rounded off to 0.5 mL.}$$

15. 4 mL grain xv = 1 g (Draw up 4 mL = grain xv.)
16. 1 mL grain $\frac{1}{320}$ = 0.2 mg (Draw up 1 mL = 0.2 mg.)
17. 0.5 mL (Draw up 0.5 mL = 0.2 mg.)
18. 1 mL 0.05 g = 50 mg (Draw up 1 mL.)
19. 1 mL 0.15 g = 150 mg (Draw up 1 mL.)
20. 1.3 mL or 21 minims (0.3 g = 300 mg, 1.3 mL = 200 mg.)
21. 0.3 mL or m v (Draw up m v = 30 units.)
22. 0.4 mL (0.01 g = 10 mg, 0.4 mL = 4 mg.)
23. 0.6 mL

$$\text{grain } \frac{1}{\underset{5}{\cancel{150}}} \times \overset{2}{\cancel{60}}\ \text{mg} = \frac{2}{5} \text{ or 0.4 mg}$$

$$\frac{0.4\ \text{mg}}{0.6\ \text{mg}} \times 1\ \text{mL} = 0.6\ \text{mL} \left(\text{Draw up 0.6 mL} = 0.4\ \text{mg or grain } \frac{1}{150}\right)$$

24. 1 mL (Draw up 1 mL = 1 : 1000 sol.)

$$0.1\% = \frac{1}{10} \div 100 = \frac{1}{10} \times \frac{1}{100} = \frac{1}{1000} \text{ or } 1 : 1000 \text{ sol}$$

25. 0.55 or 0.6 mL grain iii = 180 mg (Draw up 0.6 mL = grain iii.)

If you made no more than three errors, go on to Lesson 8. If not, solve the Additional Practice Problems with no more than three errors before proceeding.

ADDITIONAL PRACTICE PROBLEMS

Each of the following problems gives the physician's orders and the amounts in which the drugs are available. For each problem, calculate the correct dose and state answer in the following form:
Draw up 0.5 mL, which equals 8 mg, from ampule which has grain $\frac{1}{4}$ per mL.

Physician's Orders	Drug Available
1. Digotoxin 0.6 mg IM stat	Digitoxin 0.2 mg per 1-mL ampule
2. Dilaudid grain $\frac{1}{48}$ q 4 hr for pain	Hydromorphone (dilaudid) 2 mg per 1-mL ampule
3. Atropine grain $\frac{1}{100}$ plus Demerol 75 mg, both IM @ 8AM	Atropine sulfate 0.4 mg per 1-mL ampule, Meperidine hydrochloride (Demerol) 100 mg per 2-mL ampule
4. Codeine grain i (H) now	Codeine phosphate 32 mg per mL
5. Cortisone 0.05 g od	Cortisone acetate suspension 50 mg per mL
6. Cyclizine 30 mg q 4 hr prn for nausea	Cyclizine lactate 50 mg per mL
7. Ephedrine sulfate grain $\frac{3}{4}$ now	Ephedrine sulfate 0.025 g per 1-mL ampule
8. Valium 10 mg IM @ 7 AM	Diazepam (Valium) 0.05 g per 1-mL ampule
9. Epinephrine 0.2 mg q 4 hr	Epinephrine 1 : 2000 per 1-mL ampule
10. Lasix 80 mg now and repeat in 2 hr	Furosemide (Lasix) 10 mg per mL

11. Heparin 10,000 units q 8 hr   Heparin sodium 15,000 units per mL

12. Apresoline 40 mg q 6 hr   Hydralazine hydrochloride (Apresoline) 20 mg per mL

13. Isoproterenol 0.02 mg q 4 hr   Isoproterenol hydrochloride 0.2 mg per mL

14. Aminophylline grain viiss IM now   Aminophylline 0.5 g per 2-mL ampule

15. Morphine grain $\frac{1}{4}$ stat   Morphine sulfate 0.01 g per 1-mL ampule

Answers to Additional Practice Problems

1. 3 mL or 3 ampules (Draw up 3 mL = 0.6 mg.)
2. 0.6 mL. [In this problem it is probably easier to convert milligrams to grains, since grain $\frac{1}{48}$ is awkward to convert:

$$2 \text{ mg} = \frac{2}{64} = \text{grain } \frac{1}{32}$$

$$\frac{\frac{1}{48}}{\frac{1}{32}} \times 1 \text{ mL} = \frac{1}{\cancel{48}_3} \times \frac{\cancel{32}^2}{1} = \frac{2}{3} \text{ or 0.6 mL.}]$$

Answer: Draw up 0.6 mL, which equals grain $\frac{1}{48}$, and discard 0.4 mL.
3. 1.5 mL atropine sulfate and 1.5 mL meperidine
4. 2 mL or 2 ampules
5. 1 mL (0.05 g = 50 mg)
6. 0.6 mL (Draw up 0.6 mL, which = 30 mg.)
7. 2 mL or 2 ampules
8. 0.2 mL (Draw up 0.2 mL, which = 10 mg.)
9. 0.4 mL. [First, convert the ratio into units of the same system:

$$1 : 2000 \text{ solution} = 1 \text{ g per 2000 mL}$$

Then,

$$0.2 \text{ mg} = 0.0002 \text{ g}$$

$$\frac{0.0002 \text{ g}}{1 \text{ g}} \times 2000 \text{ mL} = 0.4 \text{ mL.}] \text{ (Draw up 0.4 mL, which = 0.2 mg.)}$$

10. 8 mL or 8 ampules, which = 80 mg
11. 0.6 mL (Draw up 0.6 mL, which = 10,000 units.)
12. 2 mL or 2 ampules
13. 0.1 mL or m iss, which = 0.02 mg
14. 2 mL
15. 1.5 mL (Use 2 ampules and draw up 1.5 mL = grain $\frac{1}{4}$.)

LESSON 8

Computing Dosages of Insulin

Objectives

After completing this lesson, the student will be able to:

- State the formula to use when determining insulin dosage using a calibrated syringe in minims.

- Determine the correct insulin dosage using an insulin syringe for the fourteen problems at the end of this lesson with no more than one error.

- Solve the fourteen problems at the end of this lesson with no more than one error for insulin dosage using a tuberculin syringe.

- Determine the correct insulin dosage using U-500 insulin and a U-100 insulin syringe *and* a tuberculin syringe.

The United States Pharmacopeia (USP) standardization of insulin is in units. Insulin is supplied in 10 mL vials at only U-100 and U-500 strengths. The meanings of these abbreviations are as follows:

U-100 insulin has 100 units per 1 mL solution

U-500 insulin has 500 units per 1 mL solution

There are also different kinds of insulin: Iletin (regular), protamine zinc (PZI), isophane insulin suspension (NPH), insulin zinc suspension (lente), insulin

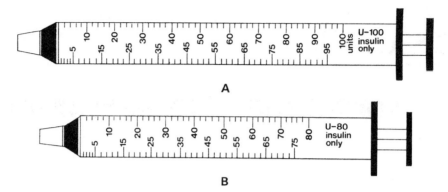

Figure 3. Insulin syringe for U-100 insulin.

zinc suspension, extended (ultralente), etc. They too are supplied in units per milliliter.

Insulin may be administered in an insulin syringe, a standard syringe, or a tuberculin syringe. If available, an insulin syringe should be used, as it is the simplest and most accurate way to measure insulin. Insulin syringes are special syringes calibrated in units (Fig. 3). The syringe most frequently used is the one for U-100 insulin.

If an insulin syringe is not available and a standard 3-cc (Fig. 4) or tuberculin syringe is used, the number of minims that will equal the units ordered must be calculated. The tuberculin syringe, which is calibrated in minims, is better for calculating small amounts of insulin (Fig. 5).

The formula for determining insulin dosage when an insulin syringe is not available is given below:

$$\frac{\text{Insulin Ordered}}{\text{Insulin on Hand}} \times 16 \text{ minims} = \text{Number Minims to Administer}$$

Insulin dosage should *not* be calculated using the value of 15 minims per milliliter, because an incorrect dose will be given.

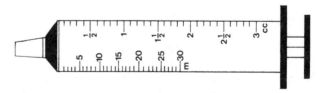

Figure 4. Standard 3-cc syringe.

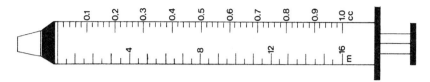

Figure 5. Tuberculin syringe.

EXAMPLE: The physician orders 90 units of Iletin (regular) U-100 insulin.

If you calculate with 15 minims rather than 16, your result will be as follows:

$$\frac{\text{Insulin Ordered}}{\text{Insulin on Hand}} \times 15 \text{ minims} = \frac{\overset{9}{\cancel{90}} \text{ units}}{\underset{2}{\cancel{100}} \text{ units}} \times \overset{3}{\cancel{15}} = \frac{27}{2}$$

$$= 13\tfrac{1}{2} \text{ minims}$$

In contrast, using 16 minims, the calculated dosage will be

$$\frac{\overset{9}{\cancel{90}} \text{ units}}{\underset{5}{\cancel{100}} \text{ units}} \times \overset{8}{\cancel{16}} = \frac{72}{5} = 14.4 \text{ minims}$$

Each minim of U-100 insulin contains $6\tfrac{1}{4}$ units of insulin; therefore, if 15 minims were used in the calculations, the patient would receive approximately 84 units instead of the 90 units ordered. In order for diabetics to maintain a relatively normal blood glucose level, they must receive the exact dosage ordered. A difference of 6 units of insulin could result in increased blood glucose levels.

A special U-100 insulin syringe has been developed for patients who use 50 units or less of U-100 insulin (Fig. 6).

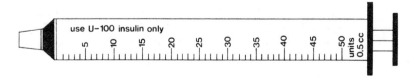

Figure 6. Special 0.5-mL insulin syringe.

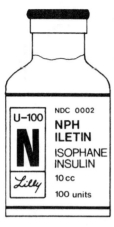

Figure 7. Vial of U-100 NPH Iletin (isophane insulin).

PROCEDURE FOR ADMINISTERING INSULIN

1. Select the insulin whose label matches the physician's order as to type and strength. For example, if the physician's order is to give 30 units of U-100 NPH Iletin insulin 30 minutes before breakfast, you would select the vial of insulin labeled NPH Iletin U-100 insulin (Fig. 7).
2. Choose the insulin syringe that matches the strength solution; ie, a syringe calibrated for U-100 insulin (Fig. 8).
3. Draw up insulin in syringe to level of units ordered by the physician.

EXAMPLE: The physician orders 30 units of NPH insulin. Label on the insulin: NPH (Isophane insulin suspension) U-100.

Answer: Select insulin that matches the physician's order, which is NPH U-100 (Fig. 7); get a U-100 insulin syringe and draw up insulin to the 30-unit mark on the syringe (Fig. 8).

The physician may also order two kinds of insulin to be given at the same time. One of these would be Iletin regular (short-acting) and the other an

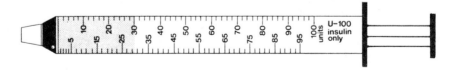

Figure 8. Insulin drawn up to 30-unit mark.

intermediate-acting (NPH, isophane insulin suspension) or longer-acting (lente, insulin zinc suspension) type.

EXAMPLE: The physician's order is, "Regular insulin 20 units with NPH insulin 32 units ac q AM (before breakfast each morning)." Label on insulin: "Regular Iletin insulin U-100," and on another vial, "Isophane insulin suspension (NPH) U-100."

Answer: Select insulin that matches physician's order and a U-100 insulin syringe, since both are U-100, and draw up 20 units of regular iletin insulin and then 32 units of NPH insulin (which would fill the syringe to the 52-unit mark).

EXAMPLE: The physician's order is, "Regular insulin 25 units and lente insulin 40 units 30 min ac. The vials are labeled, "Regular (crystalline zinc) insulin U-100" and "Lente (insulin zinc suspension) U-100." There are no U-100 insulin syringes, so a tuberculin syringe will have to be substituted. These problems are solved separately, but the insulins are administered in a single syringe.

To determine the number of minims of regular insulin, substitute in the formula:

$$\frac{\overset{}{\cancel{25}}\,U}{\underset{4}{\cancel{100}}\,U} \times \overset{4}{\cancel{16}} \text{ minims} = 4 \text{ minims (or 0.3 cc) regular insulin}$$

Determine the number of minims lente insulin in the same fashion:

$$\frac{\overset{2}{\cancel{40}}\,U}{\underset{5}{\cancel{100}}\,U} \times \cancel{16} \text{ minims} = \frac{32}{5} = 6\tfrac{2}{5} \text{ or 6.4 minims or 0.4 cc lente insulin}$$

Answer: Draw up 4 minims U-100 regular insulin in the tuberculin syringe and then draw up 6.4 minims of lente insulin for a total of 10.4 minims in the tuberculin syringe.

Occasionally diabetics are resistant to insulin, or require large doses to control their blood glucose level. U-500 insulin is given usually for doses above 100 units; therefore, the formula for determining insulin dosage utilizing a tuberculin syringe would be used, or the correct dosage would have to be calculated for a U-100 syringe.

EXAMPLE: The physician orders 350 units of Regular insulin before breakfast. Available insulin is Regular U-500. Using a tuberculin

syringe and the insulin formula:

$$\frac{\text{Insulin Ordered}}{\text{Insulin on Hand}} \times 16\ m = \frac{\overset{7}{\cancel{350}}\ \text{U}}{\underset{10}{\cancel{500}}\ \text{U}} \times 16\ m = 11.2\ m$$

Draw up 11.2 minims of U-500 Regular insulin, which = 350 units.

EXAMPLE: Using a U-100 syringe:

$$\frac{\text{Dose Ordered}}{5} = \text{Number Units of U-500 Insulin to Draw up Using a U-100}$$

(U-500 insulin is five times stronger then U-100 insulin)

Substituting in the formula:

$$\frac{\text{Dose Ordered}}{5} = \frac{350\ \text{U}}{5} = 70\ \text{units}$$

Answer: Draw up 70 units of U-500 Regular insulin (70-unit mark) on the U-100 syringe which = 350 units.

PRACTICE PROBLEMS

In your answers to the following problems, state which syringe and insulin you would select and how you would prepare the injection using an insulin syringe.

1. 35 units of NPH (isophane insulin suspension) insulin 30 minutes ac breakfast qd (30 minutes before breakfast each day). Insulin available is U-100.

2. 48 units lente insulin U-100 (insulin zinc suspension) 1 hour ac breakfast qd.

3. 40 units regular (Iletin) insulin U-100 30 minutes ac tid (30 minutes before meals 3 times a day).

4. 26 units ultralente (insulin zinc suspension, extended) U-100, 1 hour ac breakfast in AM.

5. 20 units regular (Iletin) insulin U-100 and NPH (isophane insulin suspension) 30 units U-100 30 minutes ac breakfast every AM.

6. 22 units semilente (insulin zinc suspension, prompt) U-80 $\frac{1}{2}$ hour ac breakfast qd ($\frac{1}{2}$ hour before breakfast every day).

7. 25 units regular (crystalline zinc) insulin U-100 and NPH (isophane insulin suspension) U-100 40 units $\frac{1}{2}$ hour ac breakfast qd.

8. 30 units PZI (protamine zinc insulin) U-100 and 20 units regular (Iletin) insulin U-100 30 minutes ac breakfast daily.

9. 46 units lente (insulin zinc suspension) U-100 1 hour ac breakfast daily.

10. 16 units regular (Iletin) U-100 with 30 units NPH (isophane insulin suspension) U-100 1 hour ac breakfast daily.

11–20. *Work the Problems 1 to 10 using a tuberculin syringe or standard syringe. (Answers will be in minims or tenths of a milliliter.)*

Calculate the following problems if U-500 insulin is available, using a tuberculin and also a U-100 insulin syringe.

21–24. Using a tuberculin syringe and U-500 insulin. Physician's order:

21. 300 units NPH (isophane insulin suspension)

22. 250 units Regular (Iletin)

23. 240 units semilente (insulin zinc suspension, prompt)

24. 150 units ultralente (insulin zinc suspension, extended)

25–28. Using a U-100 insulin syringe and U-500 insulin and the physician's orders in Problems 21 through 24.

Answers to Practice Problems

1. Select NPH U-100 insulin and a U-100 insulin syringe and draw up insulin to the 35-unit mark on the U-100 syringe.
2. Select lente U-100 insulin and a U-100 insulin syringe and draw up insulin to the 48-unit mark on the U-100 syringe.
3. Select regular U-100 insulin and a U-100 insulin syringe and draw up insulin to the 40-unit mark on the U-100 syringe.
4. Select ultralente U-100 insulin and a U-100 insulin syringe and draw up to the 26-unit mark on the U-100 syringe.
5. Select regular U-100 insulin and NPH U-100 insulin and a U-100 insulin syringe. Draw up regular insulin to the 20-unit mark, and then draw up NPH insulin to the 50-unit mark (30 units NPH insulin) on U-100 syringe.
6. Select semilente U-80 insulin and a U-80 insulin syringe and draw up insulin to 22-unit mark on the U-80 syringe.
7. Select regular U-100 insulin and NPH U-100 insulin and a U-100 insulin syringe. Draw up 25 units of regular insulin to 25-unit mark on syringe, then draw up NPH insulin to the 65-unit mark (40 units NPH) on U-100 syringe.
8. Select PZI (protamine zinc insulin) U-100 and regular insulin U-100. Draw up 30 units of the PZI insulin to 30-unit mark on syringe and then draw up regular insulin to 50-unit mark on U-100 syringe.
9. Select lente U-100 insulin and a U-100 insulin syringe and draw up insulin to the 46-unit mark on the U-100 syringe.
10. Select regular U-100 insulin and NPH U-100 insulin. Draw up regular insulin to the 16-unit mark on the U-100 syringe and then draw up NPH insulin to the 46-unit mark (30 units NPH insulin) on the U-100 syringe.
11. 5.6 minims or 0.3 cc of NPH U-100 insulin.

12. 7.7 minims or 0.5 cc of lente U-100 insulin.
13. 6.4 minims or 0.4 cc regular insulin.
14. 4 minims or 0.2 cc ultralente U-100 insulin.
15. 3.2 minims or 0.2 cc of regular U-100 insulin and 4.8 minims or 0.3 cc of NPH U-100 insulin. [Draw up 3 minims or 0.2 cc of regular U-100 insulin and *then* draw up (in same syringe) NPH U-100 insulin to the 8-minim or 0.5-cc mark on the syringe (5 minims or 0.3 cc of NPH insulin).]
16. 4.4 minims or 0.3 cc of semilente U-80 insulin.
17. 4 minims or 0.2 cc regular U-100 insulin and 6.4 minims or 0.4 cc of NPH U-100 insulin. (Draw up 4 minims or 0.2 cc of regular insulin and then $6\frac{1}{2}$ minims or 0.4 cc of NPH insulin to $10\frac{1}{2}$-minim or 0.6-cc mark on the tuberculin syringe.)
18. 4.8 minims of 0.3 cc of PZI U-100 insulin and 3.2 minims or 0.2 cc of regular insulin. (Draw up 5 minims or 0.3 cc of PZI and then 3 minims or 0.2 cc of regular insulin to 8-minim or 0.5-cc mark on the tuberculin syringe.)
19. 7.4 minims or 0.4 cc of lente U-100 insulin.
20. 2.6 minims or 0.2 cc regular U-100 insulin and 4.8 minims or 0.3 cc of NPH U-100 insulin.

Using the tuberculin syringe:
21. *m* 9.6. Draw up 9.6 minims of U-500 NPH insulin which equals 300 units insulin.
22. *m* 8. Draw up 8 minims of U-500 Regular insulin which equals 250 units insulin.
23. *m* 7.7. Draw up 7.7 minims U-500 semilente insulin which equals 240 units insulin.
24. *m* 4.8. Draw up 4.8 minims of U-500 ultralente insulin which equals 150 units.

Using a U-100 insulin syringe:
25. 60 units. Draw up U-500 NPH insulin to the 60-unit mark on the U-100 syringe which = 300 units.
26. 50 units. Draw up U-500 Regular insulin to the 50-unit mark on the U-100 syringe which = 250 units.
27. 48 units. Draw up semilente U-500 insulin to the 48-unit mark on the U-100 syringe which = 240 units.
28. 30 units. Draw up ultralente U-500 insulin to the 30-unit mark on the U-100 syringe which = 150 units.

If you made no more than two errors in either set of problems, go on to Lesson 9. If not, review Lesson 8 and try the problems again.

LESSON 9

Computing Dosages of Drugs in Powder Form

Objectives

After completing this lesson, the student will be able to:

- State the formula for preparing multiple-dose vials of medication in powder form.

- Solve the practice problems at the end of this lesson with no more than one error.

Penicillin and other antibiotics come in powder form in either single-dose vials or multiple-dose vials that must be reconstituted (dissolving the dry powder in a diluent to form a solution) to be administered intramuscularly or intravenously. In powder form, the penicillins will remain stable for several years, but in reconstituted form they deteriorate rapidly.

In the single-dose vials, add the amount of diluent stated on the vial, or enough diluent to dissolve the drug, usually 1 to 2 mL.

In multiple-dose vials the amount of diluent needed to dissolve the medication varies with the type and amount of drug. Directions for dissolving the drug and the amount of diluent are usually listed on the vial, on the box containing the vial, or in the informational pamphlet accompanying the drug. (Multiple-dose vials have a capacity of from 5 to 20 mL.) These directions also give the amount of drug displacement and the volume of the drug after it is in solution.

Directions: **Add 1.6 mL of sterile water which will yield 2 mL of reconstituted solution. (The drug displacement or amount of drug is 0.4 mL.)**

If the physician orders 0.5 g streptomycin sulfate (Strycin) q 6 hr IM and the vial is labeled 2 g of powder with the above directions, this problem can be solved as any dosage problem from prepared solution. Using the dosage formula and the directions above:

$$\frac{\text{Dose Ordered}}{\text{Drug on Hand}} \times \text{Dilution} = \frac{0.5 \text{ g}}{\cancel{2} \text{ g}} \times \cancel{2} \text{ mL} = 0.5 \text{ mL}$$

The vial should be labeled "0.5 g = 0.5 mL" and include the time and date the drug was reconstituted.

EXAMPLE: Give 300,000 units of penicillin G IM q 4 hr. The vial is labeled, "5,000,000 units—add 18 mL of sterile water to yield 20 mL solution."

As in the problem above, the pharmaceutical company has provided information on the amount of diluent to be added. Substituting in the formula:

$$\frac{\text{Dose Ordered}}{\text{Drug on Hand}} \times \text{Dilution} = \frac{\overset{3}{\cancel{300,000}} \text{ U}}{\underset{5}{\cancel{5,000,000}} \text{ U}} \times \overset{2}{\cancel{20}} \text{ mL} = 1.2 \text{ mL}$$

The vial would be labeled, "300,000 units = 1.2 mL."

If the pharmaceutical company does not include the instructions as to how much diluent to add, it is desirable to dissolve the drug in the amount of diluent necessary so that 0.5 or 1 cc equals the dose ordered.

Formulas for preparing penicillins and antibiotics (drugs in powder form) when the pharmaceutical company does not provide information as to amount of diluent are given below. Note that the second formula is a simplification of the first achieved by omitting a few of the mathematical steps.

FORMULAS FOR PREPARING PENICILLINS AND ANTIBIOTICS

---

1. Proportion Formula

Dose Ordered: 1 mL :: Total Amount of Drug: x

---

2. Simplified Formula

$$\frac{\text{Total Drug on Hand}}{\text{Dose Ordered}} \times 1 \text{ mL} = \text{Amount Diluent Required}$$

to Add to Vial Powder so
that Dose Ordered = 1 mL

EXAMPLE: The physician's order is, "Streptomycin sulfate (Strycin) 500 mg q 6 hr IM." Streptomycin sulfate comes in a multiple-dose vial containing 3 g of powder. Prepare this solution so that 500 mg = 1 mL.

First, milligrams must be converted to grams, or grams to milligrams: 3 g = 3000 mg. Then, substituting the values into the formula:

$$\frac{\text{Drug on Hand}}{\text{Dose Required}} \times 1 \text{ mL} = \text{Amount of Diluent (mL)} = \frac{\overset{6}{\cancel{3000}} \text{ mg}}{\underset{1}{\cancel{500}} \text{ mg}}$$

$$= \frac{6 \text{ mg}}{\text{mg}} \times 1 \text{ mL} = 6 \text{ mL}$$

Thus, 6 mL is the amount of diluent to add to make 1 mL of solution contain 500 mg streptomycin. You should then label the vial, "500 mg = 1 mL."

The formula used in the example is a simplified version of the following proportion formula:

Dose Required : 1 mL :: Drug on Hand : x (Diluent)

NOTE: The 1 mL is the standard injection amount that is desired. In theory, it could be another amount.

We can use this proportion formula to solve the above example by inserting the values given and then multiplying the extremes and then the means:

500 mg : 1 mL :: 3000 mg : x

500 mg x = 3000 mg

x = 6 mL

NOTE: The person who adds the diluent should always label the vial to indicate the number of units (mg, etc) as well as date and time drug was reconstituted.

EXAMPLE: Dilute 1,000,000 units of penicillin powder so that 400,000 units equal 1 mL, the dose ordered.

Substitute these values in the formula:

$$\frac{\text{Drug on Hand}}{\text{Dose Required}} \times 1 \text{ mL} = \text{Amount of Diluent} = \frac{\overset{5}{\cancel{1,000,000}} \text{ units}}{\underset{2}{\cancel{400,000}} \text{ units}}$$

$$= \frac{5 \text{ units}}{2 \text{ units}} \times 1 \text{ mL} = 2.5 \text{ mL}$$

Answer: Add 2.5 mL of diluent to vial containing 1,000,000 units penicillin powder so that 1 mL contains 400,000 units.

Occasionally, calculating the total volume (diluent required) so as to have 1 mL contain the dose ordered will give a result that is greater than the volume of vial. When this happens, you should use 0.5 mL in Formula 2 rather than 1 mL (which is the same as having *both* the amount of diluent and the amount to be injected).

EXAMPLE: Give 200,000 units penicillin G, IM, q 4 hr. The vial contains 3,000,000 units of powder and has a capacity of only 10 mL.

If you make your calculations using 1 mL, your answer will be 15 mL:

$$\frac{\text{Total Drug on Hand}}{\text{Dose Ordered}} \times 1 \text{ mL} = \frac{\overset{15}{\cancel{3,000,000}}}{\cancel{200,000}} \times 1 \text{ mL} = 15 \text{ mL}$$

Obviously, you cannot inject 15 mL into a 10-mL vial, so 0.5 mL should be substituted for 1 mL in the formula:

$$\frac{\overset{15}{\cancel{3,000,000}}}{\cancel{200,000}} \times 0.5 \text{ mL} = 7.5 \text{ mL}$$

The vial would then be labeled, "0.5 mL = 200,000 units." And the date and time the powder was reconstituted would, as usual, be indicated. (You might have been able to see before making the first calculation that 0.5 mL should be used since the amount of drug on hand was more than 10 times the dose ordered.)

Another situation in which it is advisable to use 0.5 mL instead of 1 mL is in calculating dosages for children. If possible, the amount of solution administered to children should be 0.5 mL, or less, since larger quantities can be more painful.

EXAMPLE: The pediatrician orders 100 mg methicillin sodium (Staphcillin) IM q 4 hr for an infant. The drug is available as 1 g of powder in a 5-mL vial.

Converting grams to milligrams and using 0.5 mL to equal the dose ordered, substitute in the formula:

$$\frac{\overset{10}{\cancel{1000}}\text{ mg}}{\cancel{100}\text{ mg}} \times 0.5 \text{ mL} = 5 \text{ mL}$$

Answer: Add 5 mL diluent and label the vial, "0.5 mL = 100 mg methicillin."

PRACTICE PROBLEMS

For each problem below, read the physician's order and label on bottle, indicate amount of diluent, and then state how vial should be labeled.

1. Pyopen 2 g IM q 6 hr. Drug available: Disodium carbenicillin (Pyopen) 5 g in powder form.

2. Staphcillin 0.5 g IM q 4 hr. Drug available: Methicillin sodium (Staphcillin) 4 g in powder form. Label instructs, "Add 5.7 mL to yield 500 mg/mL."

3. Crystalline penicillin 300,000 units IM q 4 hr. Drug available: Potassium penicillin G (Crystalline penicillin) 3,000,000 units. Instructions on label: Add 9.6 mL diluent to yield 10 mL. How would you label this vial?

4. Penicillin G 400,000 units IM q 6 hr. Drug available: Potassium penicillin G 5,000,000 units. Instructions on label:

Add Diluent	Concentration
18 mL	250,000 units per mL
8 mL	500,000 units per mL

   Which diluent would you choose and how would you label the vial?

5. Prepare a vial of drug in powder form labeled 1 g to give 125 mg per 0.3 mL.

6. How much water (sterile) would you add to a vial containing 5 g of powdered drug so the patient will receive 1000 mg per mL?

7. Prepare a vial of Cephalosporin (Keflin) which contains 1 g powder to give the patient 200 mg per mL.

8. Oxacillin 500 mg IM q 4 hr. Drug available: Oxacillin 2 g in powder form.

9. Tetracycline hydrochloride IM 100 mg q 8 hr. Drug available: Tetracycline hydrochloride 250 mg in powder form.

10. Nafcillin 500 mg IM q 4 hr. Drug available: Nafcillin sodium 4 g in powder form. Label reads: Add 5.7 mL diluent to yield 0.5 g per mL.

Answers to Practice Problems

1. Add 2.5 mL diluent. Label vial 1 mL = 2 g.
2. Follow directions given. Add 5.7 mL diluent and label vial 500 mg or 0.5 g = 1 mL.
3. Label vial 1 mL = 300,000 U. [Note that the regular dosage formula is used since you have dose ordered; dose on hand; and total amount, which is 10 mL:

$$\frac{\overset{1}{\cancel{300,000}}\ \text{U}}{\underset{10}{\cancel{3,000,000}}\ \text{U}} \times \overset{1}{\cancel{10}}\ \text{mL} = 1\ \text{mL} = 300,000\ \text{units}$$

4. Add 8 mL. 1 mL = 500,000 units. Give 0.8 mL per dose to equal 400,000 units. Label vial 0.8 mL = 400,000 units.
5. Add 2.4 mL to 1 g powder, then label vial 0.3 mL = 125 mg.
6. Add 5 mL. Label vial 1000 mg = 1 mL.
7. Add 5 mL. Label vial 1 mL = 200 mg.
8. Add 4 mL. Then label vial 1 mL = 500 mg.
9. Add 2.5 mL. Then label vial 1 mL = 100 mg.
10. Add 5.7 mL as directed. Label vial 500 mg = 1 mL.

If you made no more than one error, go on to Lesson 10. If not, solve the Additional Practice Problems with no more than one error before proceeding.

ADDITIONAL PRACTICE PROBLEMS

For each problem below, read the physician's order and label on the vial, and then indicate the amount of diluent, dosage if asked for, and how vial should be labeled.

Physician's Order

Label on Vial

1. Staphcillin 125 mg IM q 6 hr (10-lb infant)

   Methicillin sodium (Staphcillin) powder 1 g in 5-mL vial

   Prepare this solution so that 0.5 mL = 125 mg.

2. Keflin 0.1 g q 6 hr IM (2-month-old infant)

   Cephalothin sodium (Keflin) powder 1 g in 5-mL vial

   Prepare this solution so that 0.5 mL = 0.1 g.

3. Ticar 0.5 g IM q 6 hr   Ticarcillin disodium (Ticar)
                                            powder 6 g. Add 12 mL diluent.

How would you label this vial?

4. Mefoxin 500 mg IM q 4 hr   Cefoxitin sodium (Mefoxin)
                                            powder 2 g

Prepare this solution so 500 mg = 1 mL.

5. Staphcillin 500 mg IM q 4 hr   Methicillin sodium (Staphcillin)
                                            powder 1 g. Add 1.5 mL
                                            sterile water to make a total
                                            of 2 mL.

How much would you give and how would you label the vial?

6. Penicillin G 500,000 units   Potassium penicillin G 5,000,000
   q 6 hr   units powder. Add 8 mL
                                            diluent to yield 10 mL.

How would you label the vial and how much would you give?

7. Aueromycin 100 mg IM   Aureomycin 0.5 g powder

Prepare this solution so 100 mg = 1 mL.

8. Pyopen 1000 mg q 4 hr   Disodium carbenicillin (Pyopen)
                                            5 g powder

Prepare this solution so 1000 mg = 0.5 mL.

9. Tobramycin sulfate 500 mg   Tobramycin sulfate 3 g
   q 6 hr   powder

Prepare this solution so 500 mg = 1 mL.

10. Streptomycin sulfate 200   Streptomycin sulfate 1 g
    mg IM q 6 hr   powder

Prepare this solution so 200 mg = 0.5 mL.

Answers to Additional Practice Problems

1. Add 4 mL sterile water. Then label vial 0.5 mL = 125 mg.
2. Add 5 mL sterile water. Then label 0.5 mL = 100 mg.
3. Label vial 1 mL = 0.5 g.

4. Add 4 mL sterile water. Then label 1 mL = 500 mg.
5. Give 1 mL. Label vial 1 mL = 500 mg.
6. Give 1 mL. Label vial 1 mL = 500,000 units.
7. Add 5 mL sterile water. Then label 1 mL = 100 mg.
8. Add 2.5 mL diluent. Then label 1 mL = 1000 mg.
9. Add 6 mL sterile water. Label vial 1 mL = 500 mg.
10. Add 2.5 mL sterile water. Then label 0.5 mL = 200 mg.

LESSON 10

Computing Dosages for Infants and Children

Objectives

After completing this lesson, and without referring to a book except when so instructed, the student will be able to:

- State Clark's, Young's, and Fried's rules for calculating dosage for infants and children.

- Calculate infant's and children's dosage correctly when given the adult dose and age or weight of the child using the appropriate formula.

- Calculate infant's and children's dosage when the physician orders medication in milligrams per kilogram body weight.

- Determine infant's and children's dosage using the body surface area (BSA) formula and the nomogram in Figure 9 when the weight and height of the child are given.*

- Calculate infant's and children's dosage using Clark's rule based on weight, and compare answers with those obtained using the BSA formula.

- Solve problems utilizing Fried's and Young's rules and compare answers obtained with those using the BSA formula *and* Clark's rule.

- Solve practice problems at end of this chapter with no more than 2 errors.

*The student may refer to the book while doing these calculations.

Although physicians specifically order the dose for children just as they do for adults, the nurse has the moral and legal responsibility to know what constitutes proper pediatric dosage of common drugs and, therefore, must know the rules or formulas for determining children's dosage. Any adult dose of medicine ordered for a child should be questioned. (A child is defined as one who is 12 years or younger.)

FORMULAS FOR DETERMINING DOSAGES

Various formulas have been devised to determine children's dosage. Each of these formulas has limitations, since, at best, each gives only an approximate dosage. These formulas provide guidelines to assist the nurse in determining the general dosage range. The data are also useful for making a judgment about dose safety before administering to a child.

The rules discussed below are used most frequently.

Clark's Rule

This rule is based on a comparison of the child's weight, in pounds, with the average adult weight of 150 lb. This formula is generally more accurate and should be used for children who are much smaller or larger than most children of same age.

$$\frac{\text{Weight of Child}}{150} \times \text{Adult Dose} = \text{Child's Dose}$$

EXAMPLE: If the adult dose of atropine sulfate is grain $\frac{1}{150}$, what is the dose for a 50-lb child?

Substituting in the formula:

$$\frac{\text{Weight of Child}}{150} \times \text{Adult Dose} = \text{Child's Dose}$$

$$\frac{\cancel{50} \text{ lb}}{150 \text{ lb}} \times \text{grain } \frac{1}{\cancel{150}_{3}} = \frac{1}{450} \text{ grains}$$

Answer: The atropine sulfate dose for a 50-lb child is grain $\frac{1}{450}$.

Young's Rule

This formula is used for children 2 to 12 years.

$$\frac{\text{Adult Dose} \times \text{Child's Age}}{\text{Child's Age} + 12} = \text{Child's Dose}$$

EXAMPLE: If the adult dose of meperidine hydrochloride (Demerol) is 100 mg, what is the dose for an 8-year-old child?

Substitute these values into Young's formula:

$$\frac{100 \text{ mg} \times 8 \text{ yr}}{8 + 12} = \frac{\overset{40}{\cancel{800}}}{\cancel{20}} = 40 \text{ mg}$$

Fried's Rule

This formula is used to determine dosage for children under 2 years of age. The child's age is expressed in months.

$$\frac{\text{Adult Dose} \times \text{Child's Age (months)}}{150} = \text{Child's Dose}$$

EXAMPLE: If the adult dose of sulfisoxazole (Gantrisin) suspension is 1 g, what is the dose for a 15-month-old infant?

Substitute these values into Fried's formula:

$$\frac{1 \text{ g} \times 15 \text{ months}}{150} = \frac{\cancel{15}}{\underset{10}{\cancel{150}}} = \frac{1}{10} = 0.1 \text{ g}$$

Pediatric Dosage From Published Sources

Dosages for infants and children expressed in milligrams per kilogram have been previously determined for many drugs and can usually be found in the *Physician's Desk Reference* (*PDR*) and the United States Pharmacopeia as part of the description of the drugs given in those sources. Using such data, you would find the correct dosage as follows:

Drug Dose in Milligrams × Child's Weight in Kilograms = Child's Dose

---

EXAMPLE: If the child's dose is listed as 2 mg / kg, and the child weighs 11 kg, the dose would be 2 mg × 11 kg = 22 mg the dose for a child weighing 11 kg.

Body Surface Area Formula

The most accurate method of determining children's dosage is by utilizing the body surface area (BSA) formula. Estimated BSA (in square meters, m^2) is determined by using the child's height and weight and the BSA nomogram. The nomogram is used as follows: The child's height is located on the left-hand scale, and the child's weight on the right-hand scale. The BSA is then determined by using a straight edge (ruler) placed on these two points, and the point at which the straight edge transects the surface area scale gives the BSA.

EXAMPLE: If a child weighs 50 lb and is 50 inches tall, his $m^2 = 0.89$.

The BSA formula is used primarily by physicians, but nurses should be aware that it is available and that routine checking of prescribed dosages for infants and children is an integral part of the pediatric nurse's function.

The BSA formula used most frequently is the BSA short form:

$$\frac{\text{Body Surface Area of Child } (m^2) \times \text{Adult Dose}}{1.73 \text{ (accepted adult BSA)}} = \text{Infant's or Child's Dose}$$

The use of the surface area is dependent on the fact that, in relation to their weight, children have a greater surface area than adults. The surface-area-to-weight ratio varies inversely with length. Thus, the infant will have proportionately more surface area, since he or she is shorter and weighs less than an adult.

Tables have been devised which give the appropriate surface area and weight of individuals of average body dimensions, but problems still exist in estimating dosage for neonates.

Several nomograms have been developed. The West nomogram is given as an illustration (Fig. 9) and should be used in solving the practice problems at the end of this lesson.

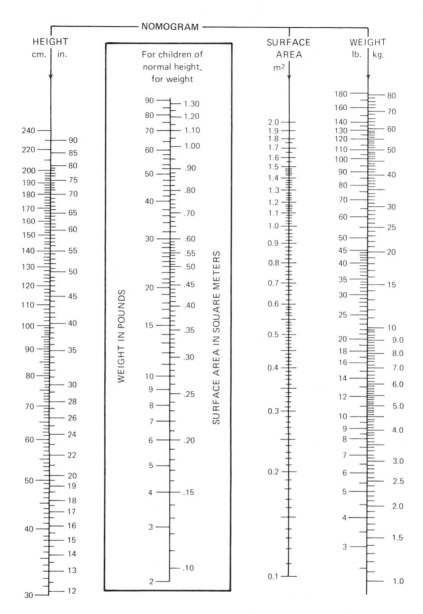

Figure 9. The West nomogram for body surface area (BSA). The BSA (in square meters, m²) is found by using a straight edge to connect a person's height (left scale) with his or her weight (right scale). The BSA is then found at the intersection of the straight edge and the surface area scale. For children of roughly average build, the boxed area may be used to find the BSA from weight alone. *(Modified from data of E. Boyd by C.D. West; from Shirkey, H.C. Drug therapy. In W.E. Nelson & V.C. Vaughn III (Eds.), Textbook of Pediatrics, 9th Ed. Philadelphia: Saunders, 1964.)*

PRACTICE PROBLEMS

Use the data in the following table to solve Problems 1 to 15 for the appropriate dosages for children. Utilize Clark's rule to make your calculations. (Make use of the West nomogram, Fig. 9, to determine the BSA.) Then complete Problems 16 to 27 as directed.

| Adult Dose | Data for Child | | | | Child's Dose (mg / kg) |
	Age	Weight (lb)	Height (in)	Weight (kg)	
1. Diazepam (Valium) 5 mg	2 yr	27	34	12.25	
2. Atropine sulfate grain $\frac{1}{150}$	18 mo	25	32	11.7	
3. Aminophylline 0.5 g	6 yr	38	42	17.4	
4. Potassium penicillin G 500,000 units	10 yr	71	50	32.3	
5. Gentamicin 80 mg	22 mo	28	33	12.7	2.5 mg/kg
6. Clindamycin phosphate (Cleocin) 200 mg	9 yr	52	48	23.6	
7. Kanamycin sulfate (Kantrex) 0.5 g	10 mo	22	29	11	7.5 mg/kg
8. Sodium Luminal (Phenobarbital sodium) grain ii	12 mo	22	31	11	3 mg/kg
9. Cephalothin sodium (Keflin) 1 g	6 mo	$12\frac{1}{2}$	25	5.7	
10. Methicillin sodium (Staphcillin) 1 g	3 mo	10	24	4.8	
11. Codeine phosphate grain i (H)	4 yr	30	40	13.65	0.5 mg/kg
12. Meperidine HCl (Demerol) 100 mg	11 yr	154	57	70	
13. Hydroxyzine HCl syrup 50 mg (10 mg/5 mL)	5 yr	32	39	14.56	
14. Milk of magnesia 30 cc	10 yr	50	50	22.2	
15. Sulfasoxazole (Gantrisin) suspension 500 mg	8 yr	48	47	21.77	

16–19. Use Fried's rule to solve Problems 2, 5, 7, and 8. Compare your answers with your results using Clark's rule and the BSA formula.

20–23. Use Young's rule to solve Problems 3, 6, 11, and 12. Compare your answers with your results using Clark's rule and the BSA formula.

24–27. Use the mg/kg body weight formula to solve Problems 5, 7, 8, and 11. (Note that the values required for the calculations given in the table are from the *Physician's Desk Reference*. As previously mentioned suitable values can also be found in the U.S. Pharmacopeia. The adult dose is not used in these calculations.)

Answers to Practice Problems

1. Clark's rule: 0.9 mg BSA formula ($m^2 = 0.55$) : 1.5 mg
2. Clark's rule: grain $\frac{1}{900}$ BSA formula ($m^2 = 0.51$) : grain $\frac{1}{500}$
3. Clark's rule: 0.126 g BSA formula ($m^2 = 0.7$) : 0.2 g
4. Clark's rule: round off 236,666 to 250,000 units BSA formula ($m^2 = 1.09$) : 315,000 units
5. Clark's rule: 15 mg BSA formula ($m^2 = 0.58$) : 27 mg
6. Clark's rule: 69 or 70 mg BSA formula ($m^2 = 0.9$) : 104 mg
7. Clark's rule: 0.07 g BSA formula ($m^2 = 0.47$) : 0.14 g
8. Clark's rule: grain $\frac{1}{3}$ BSA formula ($m^2 = 0.5$) : grain $\frac{1}{2}$
9. Clark's rule: 0.083 g BSA formula ($m^2 = 0.37$) : 0.2 g
10. Clark's rule: 0.06 g BSA formula ($m^2 = 0.28$) : 0.156 or 0.16 g
11. Clark's rule: grain $\frac{1}{5}$ BSA formula ($m^2 = 0.6$) : grain $\frac{1}{3}$. [Remember medications come in fractions with 1 for numerator most of time, so they should be reduced by dividing numerator into denominator.]
12. Clark's rule: 102 mg BSA formula ($m^2 = 1.75$) : 101 mg. [Although this is an 11-yr-old child, by weight an adult dose would probably be given.]
13. Clark's rule: 10.6 mg or 5 mL BSA formula ($m^2 = 0.65$) : 19 mg or 10 mL
14. Clark's rule: 10 cc BSA formula ($m^2 = 0.89$) : 15 cc
15. Clark's rule: 160 mg BSA formula ($m^2 = 0.85$) : 246 mg
16. grain $\frac{1}{1250}$
17. 11 mg
18. 0.03 g
19. $\frac{12}{75}$ or grain $\frac{1}{6}$

20. 0.16 g
21. 86 mg
22. grain $\frac{1}{4}$
23. 47.8 or 50 mg. [Note difference in this dosage and those derived using Clark's rule and the BSA formula.]
24. 31.75 mg
25. 82.5 mg
26. 33 mg
27. 6.8 mg

LESSON 11

Review

Objective

Having completed Lessons 1 through 10, the student should be able to:

- Solve the review problems in this lesson with no more than seven errors.

REVIEW PROBLEMS

Write as Arabic numbers:

1. XL _____   2. XIII _____   3. LXXX _____

Write as Roman numerals:

4. 45 _____   5. 33 _____   6. 50 _____

Express each of the following decimal fractions in words and then as a common fraction:

	Words	Fraction
0.03	7. _____	8. _____
0.017	9. _____	10. _____
0.5	11. _____	12. _____
0.0004	13. _____	14. _____

Express the following percents as decimal fractions and common fractions:

	Decimal Fraction	Common Fraction
100%	15. _____	16. _____
25%	17. _____	18. _____
$\frac{1}{4}$%	19. _____	20. _____
4%	21. _____	22. _____

Express the following in alternate forms:

	Decimal Fraction	Percent	Ratio
$\frac{3}{4}$	23. _____	24. _____	25. _____

	Decimal Fraction	**Percent**	**Ratio**
$\dfrac{1}{100}$	26. _____	27. _____	28. _____
$\dfrac{1}{3}$	29. _____	30. _____	31. _____
$\dfrac{1}{1000}$	32. _____	33. _____	34. _____

Arrange the following series in order of magnitude (from the largest to smallest value):

35. 0.016, 0.16, 0.106, 1.016

36. 0.041, 0.0041, 0.410, 0.0401

Arrange the following series in order, from largest to smallest value:

37. $\dfrac{1}{64}, \dfrac{1}{20}, \dfrac{1}{16}, \dfrac{1}{32}, \dfrac{1}{4}$

38. $\dfrac{3}{4}, \dfrac{5}{8}, \dfrac{5}{6}, \dfrac{2}{3}, \dfrac{5}{12}$

Convert the following amounts from the Metric to the Apothecaries' system:

39. 0.5 g = _____ grains

40. 0.0004 g = _____ grain

41. 20 mg = _____ grain

42. 5 mL = _____ minim

Convert the following amounts from the Apothecaries' to the Metric system:

43. grain $\dfrac{1}{100}$ = _____ g = _____ mg

44. grain $\dfrac{1}{2}$ = _____ mg = _____ g

45. grain v = _____ mg = _____ g

46. *m* xvi = _____ cc = _____ mL

Change grams to milligrams and milligrams to grams:

47. 0.1g = _____ mg

48. 1 g = _____ mg

49. 60 mg = _____ g   50. 1 mg = _____ g

51. The physician orders aspirin grain x po q 4 hr. The drug available is acetylsalcylic acid (aspirin) 0.3 g each. How many tablets will you give?

52. The physician orders grain lx of a medication which is labeled, "grain xx = 5 mL." How many milliliters will you give? How many drams?

53. The physician writes an order for 2400 mL of fluid to be given po in 24 hours. How many glassfuls will the patient drink in the 24 hours?

54. Billy, 6 years old, is being discharged from the hospital on erythromycin suspension 80 mg orally bid. The label states, "Erythromycin suspension 20 mg/mL." How many milliliters would Billy receive per dose? How many drams? How would you teach Billy's mother to measure the medicine at home?

55. If Billy's physician wants to see him when he has completed his medicine, when would you make the appointment in the clinic if the bottle contains ℥ i (1 oz) of the medication?

56. The physician orders 3 g of magnesium sulfate IM. The drug available is labeled, "Magnesium sulfate 50% solution, 2-mL ampule." How many milliliters would the patient receive?

57. Oxytetracycline hydrochloride (Terramycin) is available in 250-mg capsules. The physician orders 0.5 g po. How many capsules would you give?

58. What percent is a solution which has 1 g of drug per 100 mL water?

59. A premature baby is one that weighs 2500 g or less. How many pounds and ounces is this?

60. Prepare a preoperative hypodermic of meperidine hydrochloride (Demerol) 75 mg and atropine 0.4 mg. Drugs available are meperidine 100 mg per 2-mL ampule and atropine 0.6 mg per 1-mL ampule.

61. The physician orders 75 units of isophane insulin suspension (NPH) U-100 and 30 units of regular (crystalline zinc) insulin U-100 30 min ac breakfast each day. What syringe would you choose? State your answer.

62. The physician orders streptomycin 500 mg q 6 hr IM. The vial is labeled, "Streptomycin sulfate 1 g (powder form). How many milliliters of sterile water would you add so that 500 mg = 1 mL.

63. The adult dose of atropine is 0.4 mg. What would be the dose for a 20-lb child?

64. What would be the dose for a 15-month-old child if the adult dose is grain ii?

65. The physician orders Kantrex 125 mg q 8 hr. The vial is labeled, "Kanamycin sulfate (Kantrex) 0.5 g in powder form." How many milliliters would you add so that 0.5 mL = 125 mg? How would you label the vial?

66. The physician orders 230 units Regular insulin. The insulin available is Regular insulin U-500. Using a tuberculin syringe, how many minims will you give?

67. The physician orders 210 units of Regular insulin. The insulin available is Regular insulin U-500. Calculate the number of units to give using a U-100 insulin syringe.

Answers to Review Problems

1. 40   2. 13   3. 80

4. XLV   5. XXXIII   6. L

7. three one hundredths or three hundredths

8. $\frac{3}{100}$ or $\frac{1}{33}$

9. seventeen one thousandths or seventeen thousandths

10. $\frac{17}{1000}$

11. five tenths

12. $\frac{5}{10}$ or $\frac{1}{2}$

13. four ten thousandths

14. $\frac{4}{10,000}$ or $\frac{1}{2500}$

15. 1.0

16. $\frac{1}{1}$

17. 0.25

18. $\frac{1}{4}$

19. 0.0025

20. $\frac{1}{400}$

21. 0.04

22. $\dfrac{1}{25}$

23. 0.75   24. 75%

25. 3 : 4

26. 0.01   27. 1%

28. 1 : 100

29. 0.33   30. 33%

31. 1 : 3

32. 0.001   33. 0.1%

34. 1 : 1000

35. 1.016, 0.16, 0.106, 0.016

36. 0.410, 0.041, 0.0401, 0.0041

37. $\dfrac{1}{4}, \dfrac{1}{16}, \dfrac{1}{20}, \dfrac{1}{32}, \dfrac{1}{64}$

38. $\dfrac{5}{6}, \dfrac{3}{4}, \dfrac{2}{3}, \dfrac{5}{8}, \dfrac{5}{12}$

39. grain viiss

40. grain $\dfrac{1}{150}$

41. grain $\dfrac{1}{3}$

42. *m* lxxv

43. 0.0006 g = 0.6 mg

44. 32 mg = 0.032 g

45. 300 mg = 0.3 g

46. 1 cc = 1 mL

47. 100 mg

48. 1000 mg

49. 0.06 g

50. 0.001 g

51. 2 tablets. [0.3 g = grain v]

52. 15 mL, ℥ iii

53. 10 glassfuls or tumblerfuls

54. 4 mL, ℥ i. Give 1 t of erythromycin suspension twice daily.

55. 4 days

56. 6 mL [50% solution = 1 : 2 sol or 1 g per 2 cc.]

57. 2 cap

58. 1%

59. $5\frac{1}{2}$ lb

60. Demerol, $1\frac{1}{2}$ mL; atropine, *m* x

61. Since 105 units is more than 1 cc, a 2-mL syringe will have to be used. You would draw up 12 minims of isophane insulin and then draw up 5 minims of regular insulin to the 17-minim mark on the 2-mL syringe.

62. 2 mL

63. 0.05 mg

64. grain $\dfrac{1}{5}$

65. 2 mL, 0.5 mL = 125 mg

66. 7.35 minims or 7 minims. Draw up 7 *m* U-500 insulin = 230 units.

67. 42 units. Draw up U-500 insulin in U-100 insulin syringe to 42-unit mark = 210 units.

If you made no more than seven errors, go on to Lesson 12. If not, solve the Additional Review Problems with no more than seven errors before proceeding.

ADDITIONAL REVIEW PROBLEMS

Write as Arabic numbers:

1. XC _____   2. XLIX _____   3. LXXIV _____

Write as Roman numerals:

4. 101 _____   5. 9 _____   6. 60 _____

Write each of the following decimal fractions in words and then express as a common fraction.

	Words	Fraction
0.008	7. _____	8. _____
3.05	9. _____	10. _____
0.00032	11. _____	12. _____
0.016	13. _____	14. _____

Express the following percents as decimal fractions and common fractions:

	Decimal Fraction	Common Fraction
1%	15. _____	16. _____
0.5%	17. _____	18. _____
5%	19. _____	20. _____
50%	21. _____	22. _____

Express the following fractions as decimal fractions, percents, and ratios:

	Decimal Fraction	Percent	Ratio
$\frac{1}{2}$	23. _____	24. _____	25. _____
$\frac{1}{50}$	26. _____	27. _____	28. _____

$\dfrac{1}{200}$ 29. ———   30. ———   31. ———

$\dfrac{5}{8}$ 32. ———   33. ———   34. ———

35. The physician orders calcium gluconate grain v IM. The drug available is labeled, "Calcium gluconate 10% solution." How much would you give?

Arrange in the following series order, from largest to smallest value:

36. 0.012, 0.124, 0.1, 0.045, 0.145

37. 0.03, 0.325, 0.3, 0.34, 0.3564

Arrange in order, from largest to smallest value:

38. $\dfrac{1}{75}, \dfrac{1}{100}, \dfrac{1}{200}, \dfrac{1}{150}$ 39. $\dfrac{9}{20}, \dfrac{4}{5}, \dfrac{3}{4}, \dfrac{9}{10}, \dfrac{1}{2}$

Convert the following amounts from the Metric to the Apothecaries' system:

40. 16 mg = ———— grain   41. 0.5 mL = ———— minim

42. 0.03 g = ———— grain   43. 0.4 mg = ———— grain

Convert the following amounts from the Apothecaries' to the Metric system:

44. grain $\dfrac{1}{6}$ = ———— g = ———— mg

45. grain viiss = ———— mg = ———— g

46. grain $\dfrac{3}{4}$ ———— mg = ———— g

47. grain xv = ———— mg = ———— g

Change grams to milligrams and milligrams to grams:

48. 0.0004 g = ———— mg   49. 0.01 g = ———— mg

50. 1000 mg = ———— g   51. 0.2 mg = ———— g

52. Prepare an intramuscular injection of grain iv from a 25% solution.

53. If a solution contains grain $\frac{1}{30}$ of drug/mL, how many minims would you give for grain $\frac{1}{120}$?

54. An infant weighs 4500 g at birth. How many pounds and ounces does the baby weigh? (This is calculated using 16 oz = 1 lb.)

55. The physician orders sodium (Prostaphlin) 500 mg IM q 6 hr. The drug available is labeled, "Oxacillin sodium 2 g in powder form." How many milliliters will you add so that 500 mg = 1 mL?

56. The physician orders 50 units of PZI U-100 insulin and 20 units of regular insulin U-100 30 minutes ac breakfast daily. State how you would prepare this injection using an insulin syringe. The insulin available is protamine zinc insulin U-100 and regular insulin U-100.

57. The physician orders penicillin G 500,000 units IM q 8 hr. The drug available is labeled: "Potassium penicillin G 2,000,000 units in powder form." How many milliliters will you add so that 500,000 U equals 1 mL?

58. The adult dose of ephedrine is grain $\frac{3}{4}$. What should be the dose for a 50-lb child?

59. The adult dose of aminophylline is 0.5 g. What should be the dose for a 12-month-old infant?

60. What percent is a solution which has grain xv of drug per 100 mL water?

61. Jimmy, a 2-year-old, is being discharged from the hospital. The physician wants him to continue taking ferrous sulfate (Feosol Elixir) 220 mg tid. The elixir is labeled, "Ferrous sulfate elixir 220 mg/5 mL." How many drams would Jimmy receive for each dose? How would you instruct his mother to give Jimmy the elixir at home?

62. The physician told Jimmy's mother to continue the ferrous sulfate until all of it had been taken. It comes in a 12-fl oz bottle. How many days will Jimmy have to take the elixir?

63. The physician orders Sodium Luminal grain iii (H) now. The drug available is labeled, "Phenobarbital sodium (Sodium Luminal) 120 mg/mL." How many milliliters should be given?

64. The physician orders penicillin 400,000 units q 6 hr. The drug available is

labeled, "Penicillin 1,000,000 per 5 mL." How many milliliters should be given?

65. The physician orders Premarin 0.00125 g od. Tablets of conjugated estrogen (Premarin) are labeled 2.5, 1.25, and 0.625 mg. Which would you order and how many would you give per dose?

66. The physician's order is 250 units of Regular insulin. Insulin available is Regular U-500. Prepare this injection using a U-100 insulin syringe.

67. Utilizing the physician's order in Problem 66 and the U-500 available insulin, prepare this injection using a tuberculin syringe. (Answer will be in minims.)

Answers to Additional Review Problems

1. 90   2. 49   3. 74
4. CI   5. IX   6. LX

7. eight thousandths   8. $\dfrac{8}{1000}$ or $\dfrac{1}{125}$

9. three and five one-hundredths   10. $\dfrac{305}{100}$

11. thirty two one hundred   12. $\dfrac{32}{100,000}$ or $\dfrac{1}{3125}$
    thousandths

13. sixteen thousandths   14. $\dfrac{16}{1000}$ or $\dfrac{1}{62}$

15. 0.01   16. $\dfrac{1}{100}$

17. 0.005   18. $\dfrac{1}{200}$

19. 0.05   20. $\dfrac{1}{20}$

21. 0.5   22. $\dfrac{1}{2}$

23. 0.5   24. 50%   25. 1 : 2
26. 0.02   27. 2%   28. 1 : 50
29. 0.005   30. $\frac{1}{2}$%   31. 1 : 200
32. 0.625   33. 62.5%   34. 5 : 8

35. Give 3.3 mL [10% solution = 1 : 10 or 1 g per 10 mL]

36. 0.145, 0.124, 0.1, 0.045, 0.012
37. 0.3564, 0.34, 0.325, 0.3, 0.03

38. $\dfrac{1}{75}$, $\dfrac{1}{100}$, $\dfrac{1}{150}$, $\dfrac{1}{200}$

39. $\dfrac{9}{10}$, $\dfrac{4}{5}$, $\dfrac{3}{4}$, $\dfrac{1}{2}$, $\dfrac{9}{20}$

40. grain $\dfrac{1}{4}$

41. *m* viii

42. grain $\dfrac{1}{2}$

43. grain $\dfrac{1}{150}$

44. 0.01 g = 10 mg. [This should have been worked by converting to milligrams first and then moving the decimal point three places to left.]
45. 500 mg = 0.5 g
46. 48 mg (50 mg) = 0.05 g. [The pharmaceutical company will label this 50 mg and 0.05 g.]
47. 1000 mg = 1 g. [This comes from your table; 900 mg is incorrect.]

48. 0.4 mg

49. 10 mg

50. 1 g

51. 0.0002 g

52. Give 16 *m* or 1 mL.
53. *m* iv
54. 9 lb, 14 oz. [4500 g = 4.5 kg (move decimal point three places to left since 1000 g = 1 kg). Then, 2.2 lb = 1 kg, so 4.5 kg × 2.2 lb = 9.9 lb or 9 lb, 14 oz.]
55. Add 4 mL. Then label 1 mL = 500 mg.
56. Choose PZI U-100 insulin and regular insulin U-100 and an U-100 insulin syringe. Draw up PZI U-100 insulin to the 50-unit mark on the U-100 syringe, and then draw up regular insulin to the 70-unit mark (20 units of regular insulin). (Total 70 units.)
57. Add 4 mL. Then label 500,000 units = 1 mL.
58. grain $\dfrac{1}{4}$
59. 0.04 g
60. 1%
61. ℥ i. Take 1 teaspoonful three times a day.
62. 24 days. [360 mL total ÷ 15 mL per day = 24 days.]
63. 1.5 mL
64. 2 mL. [This is a regular dosage problem, since there is an amount ordered and an amount in a given solution.]
65. Choose 1.25-mg tablets, which equal 0.00125 g each, and give 1 tablet a day.
66. 50 units of U-500 to 50-unit mark on U-100 syringe.
67. 8 minims. Draw up 8 *m* U-500 insulin = 250 units.

LESSON 12

Calculating the Flow Rate for Intravenous Infusions

Objectives

After completing this lesson and without referring to a book except where indicated, the student will be able to:

- Write the formula for determining the flow rate (drops per minute) when the drop factor and the milliliters per minute are given.

- Write the formula for determining the flow rate for the total volume ordered when the drop factor and the total time of administration are given.

- Compute the flow rate when the drop factor and the milliliters per minute are given.

- Compute the flow rate of an infusion when the total volume, drop factor, and total time desired for the infusion to be administered are given.

- Compute the flow rate of an infusion for an infant or young child when given the drop factor, total volume to be administered, and the total time for administration.

- Calculate the flow rate for infusions while referring to Table 4 for converting weight to body surface area and the formula for determining the flow rate using body surface area (m^2), shown on page 139.*

*These calculations may be made while looking at your book.

- Check the correctness of a fluid-therapy order by using the table for converting weight to surface area and the rules for calculating IV fluids using the body surface area, given on pages 138 and 139.*

- Solve the practice problems at the end of this lesson with no more than four errors.

CONSIDERATIONS IN FLUID ADMINISTRATION

Ideally, when physicians order intravenous (IV) fluids, they should also designate how fast they wish the infusion to be given; ie, either how many milliliters per minute or the total length of time for the infusion to be administered. Some physicians indicate only the type and amount of fluid to be given in their orders, and the nurse has to determine the flow rate. When the nurse receives the order for fluids, the physician should be asked to write how fast the infusion should be given.

Factors Affecting Infusion Rate

There are many factors that will influence the rate at which an infusion should be administered. Some of these are as follows[†]:

Factor	Consideration
1. Type of fluid	A 5% dextrose solution can be administered faster than 10% dextrose or 5% alcohol.
2. Need for fluids	The patient who is dehydrated or hemorrhaging can take fluids faster and in larger amounts.
3. Cardiac or renal status	The heart and kidneys play a major role in utilization of fluids; therefore, if the pumping action of the heart is inadequate or the kidneys are not excreting properly, rapid or excessive amounts of fluid could cause dangerous excesses.
4. Body size	The body surface area is an important criterion for fluid infusion rate and water and electrolyte requirements, since it provides a quantitative index of total metabolic activity. (Short obese persons have proportionately less body surface area than tall, thin persons.)

---

*Metheny, N. & Snively, W. D. *Nurses' Handbook of Fluid Balance*, 4th Ed. Philadelphia: Lippincott, 1983, p. 143.
[†] Metheny, N. & Snively, W. D., *op. cit.*, p. 144.

5. Age

The aged almost always have some degree of cardiac or renal impairment; therefore, fluids are administered more slowly to them than to young adults.

6. Patient's reaction

The patient's reaction to the infusion is also a good guide in determining the flow rate. If he is restless, has difficulty breathing, and so forth, the flow rate may need to be decreased.

7. Size of the vein

Mechanical factors that influence the gravity flow rate include the following*:

1. Change in needle position (needle against vein wall).
2. Height of infusion bottle.
3. Patency of needle (blood clot in needle may slow rate).
4. Limb movement or exercise.
5. Venous spasm.
6. Plugged air vent.
7. Condition of final filter.
8. Crying in infants.

Patients with high fever, liver disease, bleeding tendencies, acidosis, thromboembolic disease, or cardiovascular disease should be observed very closely when receiving infusions.

Body Surface Area

As stated previously, the body surface area (BSA) is an important criterion for determining the flow rates of infusions. It can also provide nurses with a simple, rapid method of checking the correctness of parenteral fluid orders, especially in regard to volume and rate of administration. Table 4 shows the approximate BSAs for individuals with average body builds.

EXAMPLE: Calculate the flow rate for a person weighing 100 lb.

Table 4 shows that a 100-lb person has a BSA of 1.4 m². Using this value and the

---

*Metheny, N. & Snively, W. D., *op. cit.*, p. 19.

TABLE 4. BODY SURFACE AREA IN SQUARE METERS FOR PERSONS
WITH AVERAGE BODY BUILDS

Weight (lb)	BSA (m²)	Weight (lb)	BSA (m²)
4	0.15	70	1.10
6	0.20	80	1.21
10	0.27	90	1.33
15	0.36	100	1.40
20	0.45	125	1.60
30	0.60	150	1.75
40	0.72	175	2.00
50	0.87	200	2.20
60	0.97	250	2.70

(Adapted from Metheny, N. & Snively, W. D. Nurses' Handbook of Fluid Balance, 4th Ed. Philadelphia: Lippincott, 1983, p. 19.)

usual rate of infusion of 3 mL per m², calculate as follows:

$$3 \text{ mL} \times m^2 = \text{Flow rate (mL/min)}$$

$$3 \text{ mL} \times 1.4 = 4.2 \text{ mL per minute}$$

There are various methods for determining the BSA, but clinicians usually employ simple nomograms that enable one to estimate rapidly the BSA from the height and body weight or from the weight alone. The BSA gauge for dosage is especially useful for checking the correctness of the amounts of water and electrolytes ordered for patients with body fluid disturbances.[*]

RULES FOR USING BSA IN CALCULATING INFUSIONS[*]

The usual flow rate for an IV infusion is 3 mL per square meter (m²) per minute.[†] However, several physiological conditions require modifications of this usual flow rate. The list below presents the rules to follow in such cases[‡]:

---

[*]Metheny, N. & Snively, W. D., op. cit., p. 19.
[†]Ibid.
[‡]Ibid.

Condition	Daily Allowable Infusion
1. Maintenance administration	1500 mL per m^2 BSA
2. Correction of moderate extracellular fluid deficit plus maintenance	2400 mL per m^2
3. Correction of severe fluid deficit plus maintenance	3000 mL per m^2
4. Replacement of concurrent fluid losses	Appropriate replacement solution on a volume-for-volume basis
5. Usual rate, except when giving initial hydrating solutions	3 mL per m^2

Since there are rules for calculating the amount of IV fluids needed based on BSA (in m^2) under various physiological conditions and the usual flow rate for an infusion is 3 ml per m^2, the nurse can check the accuracy of daily therapy orders by making use of the following formula:

$$\text{Recommended Infusion (mL)} \times \text{BSA (m}^2\text{)} = \begin{array}{l}\text{Total Amount} \\ \text{of Fluid per Day}\end{array}$$

EXAMPLE: The physician orders 3400 mL to be given over a period of 24 hours to a 110-lb boy with a moderate fluid deficit.

Table 4 shows that a 110-lb boy has a BSA of 1.5 m^2. Rule 2 above says that the amount of fluid needed to correct a moderate deficit is 2400 mL per m^2 per day. Substituting these values in the formula given, we have the following:

$$\text{Recommended infusion} \times \text{m}^2 = \text{Total fluid}$$

$$2400 \text{ mL} \times 1.5 \text{ m}^2 = 3600 \text{ mL}$$

Thus, 3400 mL would be the correct amount to be given in 24 hours to this boy.
   The formula presented below shows how to calculate the flow rate for adults using the knowledge of BSA.

$$\text{Standard Flow (3 mL)} \times \text{BSA (m}^2\text{)} = \text{Flow Rate (mL/min)}$$

EXAMPLE: Calculate the flow rate for the boy in the previous problem:

$3 \text{ mL} \times 1.5 \text{ m}^2 = 4.5 \text{ mL}$ per minute

The next formula shows how to calculate the flow rate in drops per minute for adults when you know the BSA.

Standard Flow (3 mL) × BSA (m²) × Drop Factor = Drops per Minute

---

EXAMPLE: For the 110-lb boy of the previous examples, calculate the flow rate in drops per minute if the drop factor is 10 drops per mL.

$3 \text{ mL} \times 1.5 \times 10 = 45$ drops per minute

CALCULATING THE FLOW RATE FOR ADMINISTRATION OF PARENTERAL FLUIDS

The rate at which fluids are given intravenously is measured in drops per minute.* This is called the *flow rate*. In order to determine the number of drops per minute, the nurse must know the drop factor for the set being used. The drop factor varies with different commercial sets and is therefore an important determinant of the flow rate, or the number of drops per minute the solution is to be infused. The *drop factor* is the number of drops the administration set delivers per milliliter of liquid and is determined by the size of the drops. For example, one commercial set may deliver 15 drops per mL, while another may deliver only 10 drops per mL. (Note that the drop factor is usually indicated on the set.)

The following list gives the drop factors (or microdrops per milliliter) for a number of commercially available infusion sets:[†]

Supplier	Regular	Pediatric	Special
Abbot	15 drops	60 microdrops	10 (blood)
McGaw	15 drops	60 microdrops	12 (blood)
Travenol	10 drops	50 microdrops (minimeter) 60 microdrops (metal drop system)	

---

*Children's IV fluids are administered in microdrops.
[†] Metheny, N. & Snively, W. D., *op. cit.,* p. 144.

The formula for determining the flow rate when given the drop factor is as follows:

> Drop Factor × Milliliters per Minute = Flow Rate (drops/min)

EXAMPLE: The physician orders an infusion to deliver 2 mL per minute and the IV set delivers 10 drops per mL. Determine the flow rate in drops per minute.

Substitute the values given into the formula and solve:

Drop Factor × Milliliters = Flow Rate

10 (drop factor) × 2 mL = 20 drops per minute

EXAMPLE: Administer the same amount of fluid with a set that delivers 15 drops per mL.

Proceed as above:

15 (drop factor) × 2 mL = 30 drops per minute

NOTE: In both examples the patient is to receive 2 mL per minute; however, as a result of the difference in drop factor, the set with a drop factor of 10 would require a flow rate of 20 drops per minute, whereas the set with a factor of 15 requires a flow rate of 30 drops per minute.

Frequently, the nurse must calculate the number of drops per minute the patient should receive so that at the end of a period of time a set amount of fluid has been given.

EXAMPLE: The physician's order is for 1000 mL of 5% dextrose in water (D / W) to be administered in 5 hours. The drop factor is 15.

The nurse must make the following series of calculations:

1. Determine the number of minutes the infusion is to run:

    5 hr × 60 min = 300 minutes

2. Determine the number of milliliters the patient is to receive per minute (use the formula below):

    $$\frac{\text{Milliliters Ordered}}{\text{Minutes to Flow}} = \text{Milliliters per Minute}$$

    $$\frac{1000 \text{ mL}}{300 \text{ min}} = 3.3 \text{ or } 3 \text{ mL per minute}$$

3. Determine the number of drops per minute required:

$$15 \text{ (drop factor)} \times 3 \text{ (mL/min)} = 45 \text{ drops per minute}$$

The formula for solving this type of problem is then as follows:

$$\frac{\text{Total of Fluid to Give}}{\text{Total Time (minutes)}} \times \text{Drop Factor} = \text{Flow Rate (drops/min)}$$

EXAMPLE: Infuse 1000 mL 5% D / W in 2 hours with an administration set with a drop factor of 10.

Substitute into the formula given above:

$$\frac{\text{Total Fluid}}{\text{Total Time}} \times \text{Drop Factor} = \text{Flow Rate}$$

$$\frac{1000 \text{ mL}}{\underset{12}{\cancel{120} \text{ min}}} \times \cancel{10} = 83 \text{ or (rounding off) } 80 \text{ drops per minute}$$

FLOW RATES FOR INFANTS

Since infants and young children are given much smaller amounts of medications than adults, the rate of flow for an infant is measured in *microdrops per minute*. Most of the sets used to give intravenous infusions to children deliver 60 microdrops per mL. The same formula as just given above is used to determine microdrops for infants, the flow rate in infants, except that microdrop replaces drop (always check the drop factor used in the agency where you work):

$$\frac{\text{Total Volume (mL)}}{\text{Total Infusion Time (min)}} \times \frac{\text{Drop Factor}}{\text{(microdrops/mL)}} = \frac{\text{Flow Rate}}{\text{(microdrops/min)}}$$

EXAMPLE: Give 100 mL of 10% D / W intravenously in 4 hours. Assume a drop factor of 60 microdrops per mL.

Substitute the values given in the formula above:

$$\frac{\text{Total Volume}}{\text{Total Infusion Time}} \times \text{Drop Factor} = \text{Flow Rate}$$

$$\frac{\overset{25}{\cancel{100} \text{ mL}}}{\underset{4}{\cancel{240} \text{ min}}} \times \cancel{60} \text{ microdrops} = 25 \text{ microdrops per minute}$$

CALCULATING TOTAL TIME TO ADMINISTER AN INFUSION

Sometimes when a physician orders IV medication, he or she specifies the rate at which it is to be administered. In the following example the nurse must calculate the length of time the infusion is to run.

EXAMPLE: Give 1000 mL normal saline at the rate of 50 drops per minute. The drop factor is 10 drops per mL.

1. Determine total number of drops ordered:

   Total Infusion (mL) × Drop Factor = Total Number of Drops

   1000 mL × 10 drops = 10,000 drops

2. Determine number of minutes medication is to flow:

   $$\frac{\text{Total Number of Drops}}{\text{Number of Drops per Minute}} = \text{Number of Minutes of Flow}$$

   $$\frac{10,000 \text{ drops}}{50 \text{ drops/min}} = 200 \text{ min}$$

3. Convert minutes to hours and minutes:

   $$\frac{200 \text{ min}}{60 \text{ min}} = 3 \text{ hr } 20 \text{ min}$$

Formula for Total Infusion Time

$$\frac{\text{Total Drops to Be Infused}}{\text{Flow Rate (drops/min)} \times 60} = \begin{array}{l}\text{Total Infusion Time} \\ \text{(in hours and minutes)}\end{array}$$

NOTE: If the drop factor is 60 guttae per mL, the flow rate per hour will be the same as the drop factor per minute (60 guttae/min) since the ratio of drops to minutes is 1 : 1.

EXAMPLE: Administer 1000 mL Ringer's lactate over a period of 10 hours, using an infusion set that delivers 60 drops per milliliter.

Flow rate for 1 hour would be:

$$\frac{\overset{100}{\cancel{1000}} \text{ mL}}{\cancel{10} \text{ hr}} = 100 \text{ mL/hr}$$

or, 100 drops per minute.

Or, using the formula:

$$\text{Flow Rate} = \frac{\text{Total Volume (mL)}}{\text{Total Infusion Time (min)}} \times \text{Drop Factor (drops/mL)}$$

$$= \frac{\overset{100}{\cancel{1000}} \text{ mL}}{\underset{10}{\cancel{600}} \text{ min}} \times \cancel{60} \text{ (drop factor)} = 100 \text{ drops/min}$$

If the drop factor is 10, 15, 20, 30 (numbers that divide evenly into 60), the same short formula may be used.

PRACTICE PROBLEMS

1. The physician orders 1000 mL Ringer's lactate to be administered in 4 hours and the drop factor is 10 drops per milliliter. Determine the following:
   a. The number of minutes the medication is to flow.
   b. The number of milliliters the patient will receive per minute.
   c. The number of drops the patient will receive per minute.

2. Give 800 mL of 10% dextrose in 6 hours. The drop factor is 15 drops per mL.
   a. Determine the total number of minutes medication is to flow.
   b. Determine the number of milliliters patient will receive per minute.
   c. Determine the number of drops per minute.

3. Give 1000 mL 5% D/W at 60 drops per minute. The drop factor is 15.
   a. Determine the total number drops to be given.
   b. Determine the total number of minutes medication is to flow.
   c. Determine the total time for infusion in hours and minutes.

4. Give 1000 mL Ringer's lactate followed by 1000 mL 10% D/W during the next 12 hours. The drop factor for the Ringer's lactate is 15, and for the dextrose, 10 drops mer mL. Allow 6 hours for each infusion. Determine the following:
   a. The number of minutes Ringer's lactate is to flow.
   b. The number of milliliters per minute for Ringer's lactate.
   c. The flow rate for Ringer's lactate.
   d. The total number minutes for dextrose to run.
   e. The number of milliliters per minute for dextrose.
   f. The flow rate for dextrose.

5. Determine the flow rate of an IV infusion for an adult if the physician ordered 1000 mL to be given in 2 hours and the drop factor is 10.

6. An adult patient was given 1000 mL normal saline in 5 hours. What was the rate of administration (flow rate) if the drop factor was 15?

7. Determine the flow rate for an IV infusion of 1200 mL to be given at rate of 3 mL per min. The drop factor is 15.

8. Determine the total length of time an IV infusion of 1000 mL will run if the patient is receiving 40 drops per minute and the drop factor is 10.

9. Give an infusion of 1000 mL 10% D/S at 35 drops per minute. Assume the drop factor is 10. What is total length of time the infusion should run?

10. Determine the flow rate of 1000 mL of leverterenol (Levophed) solution to be run at rate of 1 mL per minute. The drop factor is 10 drops per mL.

11. Give an infant a 100-mL infusion at a flow rate of 30 microdrops per minute. Assume the drop factor is 60 microdrops per mL.
    a. Determine the total number of microdrops to be given.
    b. Determine the total number of minutes the IV solution is to flow.
    c. Determine the total number hours and minutes the IV solution is to flow.

12. Give an infant a 90-mL IV infusion at rate of 30 microdrops per minute. Assume a drop factor of 60.
    a. Determine the total number microdrops to be given.
    b. Determine the total number of minutes infusion is to flow.
    c. Determine the total number hours and minutes the solution is to flow.

13. If the physician orders 90 mL of medication to be administered over a period of 8 hours to an infant, and the drop factor is 60 microdrops per mL, what should the flow rate be?

14. Give an infant 60 mL of IV solution at 0.5 cc per minute. The drop factor is 60.
    a. Determine the total number of microdrops.
    b. Determine the total number of minutes of flow.
    c. Determine the hours and minutes the solution is to flow.
    d. Determine the flow rate.

15. Give a 125-mL infusion over a period of 12 hours. The drop factor is 60. What should the flow rate be?

Answers to Practice Problems

1. a. 240 minutes to flow
   b. 4 mL per minute
   c. 40 drops per minute (flow rate)
2. a. 360 minutes
   b. 2 mL per minute
   c. 30 drops per minute
3. a. 15,000 drops to be given
   b. 250 minutes to flow
   c. 4 hours and 10 minutes
4. a. 360 minutes Ringer's lactate is to flow
   b. 3 mL per minute

    c. 45 drops per minute for Ringer's lactate

    d. 360 minutes for dextrose to flow

    e. 3 mL per minute

    f. 30 drops per minute for dextrose

5. Flow rate would be 8.3 mL round off to 8 mL or 83 drops per minute round off to 80 drops per minute.

6. Flow rate was 50 drops per minute, or 3.3 mL per minute.

7. 45 drops per minute

8. 4 hours and 10 minutes

9. 4 hours and 45 minutes

10. Flow rate would be 10 drops per minute.

11. a. 6000 microdrops to be given

    b. 200 minutes to flow

    c. 3 hours and 20 minutes

12. a. 5400 total microdrops

    b. 180 minutes

    c. 3 hours

13. 11 or 12 microdrops per minute

14. a. 3600 microdrops (total)

    b. 120 minutes (total)

    c. 2 hours

    d. 30 microdrops per minute

15. Flow rate would be 10 or 11 microdrops per minute.

If you made no more than four errors, go on to Lesson 13. If not, solve the Additional Practice Problems before proceeding.

ADDITIONAL PRACTICE PROBLEMS

Use the BSA table based on weight on p. 138, the list of physiological conditions to determine daily fluid needs on p. 139 and the formula for calculating flow rate using BSA (m^2) on p. 139 to solve the following six problems.

1. The physician orders 3000 mL of fluid to be given over a period of 24 hours to a 50-lb child with a moderate fluid deficit. Determine the following:

    a. If this is the correct amount.

    b. Flow rate of the infusion (in mL/min).

(Use the BSA table based on weight, p. 138, and the formula for calculating flow rates, p. 139.)

2. What would be the approximate flow rate per hour of the above infusion?

3. A patient with a severe fluid deficit had 8000 mL ordered over a period of 8 hours. The weight of the patient was 115 lb.
   a. Determine if this was the correct amount for this patient.
   b. What should the flow rate be (in mL/min)?

4. A 10-lb infant with a moderate fluid deficit had 1000 mL of fluids ordered over a 24-hour period. Determine the following:
   a. If this was the correct amount.
   b. The flow rate (in mL/min).

5. Determine the flow rate (in mL/min) for the administration of 2400 mL over 24 hours for an 80-lb child with moderate fluid deficit. Was this the correct amount?

6. A 250-mL maintenance infusion is ordered for a premature infant weighing 4 lb. The total infusion is to be administered in 24 hours. Determine the following:
   a. If this is the correct amount.
   b. What the flow rate (mL/min) should be.
   c. How many milliliters per hour the baby should receive.

Answers to Additional Practice Problems

1. a. Incorrect amount. [The BSA for a 50-lb child is 0.87 m^2. The amount of fluid to be given during moderate deficit is 2400 mL $\times$ m^2 : 2400 $\times$ 0.87 = 2088. Thus, 2088 mL or 2000 mL would be the correct amount.]
   b. 1.3 mL per minute. $\dfrac{2000 \text{ mL}}{1440 \text{ min}} = 1.3 \text{ mL}$
2. 78 mL per hour.
3. a. Incorrect amount. [In cases of severe fluid deficit, 3000 mL per square meter of BSA should be given per 24 hours. A 115-lb individual has a BSA of 1.5 m^2. Then, 3000 $\times$ 1.5 = 4500. The correct amount would be 4500 mL per day.]
   b. 4.5 mL per minute.
4. a. Incorrect amount. [The BSA for a 10-lb infant is 0.27 m^2; fluid amount in moderate deficit would be 2400 mL per day. Thus, correct amount would be: 2400 $\times$ 0.27 = 648 mL or 600 mL.]
   b. 0.42 mL per minute.

5. Flow rate: 2 mL per minute. [Total fluid was incorrect. An 80-lb child would have a BSA of 1.21 m^2. Under conditions of moderate fluid deficit, 2400 mL per day × m^2 is recommended. Thus, the correct amount would be: 2400 × 1.21 = 2904 mL.]

6. a. Incorrect amount. [A 4-lb baby's BSA is 0.15 m^2. The recommended maintenance infusion is 1500 mL × m^2. Thus, 1500 × 0.15 = 225 mL per 24 hours is correct.]

   b. 0.15 mL per minute.

   c. 9 mL per hour.

LESSON 13

Calculating Intravenous Medications

Objectives

After completing this lesson, and without referring to a book, the student will be able to:

- Write the formula for determining the flow rate for intravenous medications when the infusion time, amount of medication, and drop factor are given.

- Write the formula for determining the flow rate when a prescribed amount of medication is ordered per minute.

- Write the formula for determining the flow rate when a prescribed amount of medication per kilogram body weight is ordered per minute.

- Calculate the flow rate for intravenous medications when infusion time, amount of medication and solution, and drop factor are given.

- Calculate the flow rate when a prescribed amount of medication is ordered per minute.

- Calculate the amount of medication a patient is receiving per minute when the total amount of medication, solution, and prescribed time period are given.

- Calculate the flow rate for a prescribed amount of intravenous medication per kilogram body weight per minute.

- Solve the practice problems at the end of this lesson with no more than three errors.

INTRAVENOUS MEDICATIONS

Medications in a specific amount of fluid are prescribed frequently to be administered intravenously over a specified time period. The flow rate for these medications is calculated in the same manner as for intravenous infusions.

The formula presented below shows how to determine flow rate for intravenous medications when infusion time, amount of medication, and drop factor are given.

$$\frac{\text{Total Volume (mL)}}{\text{Total Infusion Time}} \times \text{Drop Factor} = \text{Flow Rate (drops/min)}$$

EXAMPLE: Infuse Velosef 1 g in 100 mL solution intravenously over a 30-minute period. The drop factor is 10 drops per mL.

Substituting in the formula:

$$\frac{100 \text{ mL}}{\underset{3}{30} \text{ min}} \times 10 \text{ (drop factor)} = 33 \text{ drops/min} \\ \text{(flow rate)}$$

In some situations, a patient may require a continuous infusion of a prescribed concentration of medication. The nurse may have to calculate the flow rate so that the patient will receive a prescribed amount of medication per minute, or she may have to calculate the quantity of medication per kilogram of body weight per minute.

The formula for determining flow rate when prescribed amount of medication is ordered per minute is as follows:

Formula 1

$$\frac{\text{Total Volume (mL)} \times \text{Drop Factor}}{\text{Total Amount Medication}} \times \text{Dose Ordered per Minute} = \text{Flow rate}$$

Or, the proportion formula may be used:

Formula 2

Total Amount Medication : Total Amount Solution :: Dose Ordered : x

Substituting in Formula 1: (Convert 0.5 g to mg = 500 mg)

$$\frac{\overset{2}{\cancel{200}} \text{ mL} \times \overset{12}{\cancel{60}} \text{ guttae}}{\underset{5}{\cancel{500}} \text{ mg}} \times 2 \text{ mg} = 48 \text{ microdrops/min} = \text{flow rate}$$

Substituting in Formula 2:*

500 mg : 200 mL :: 2 mg : x

500 x = 400

x = 0.8 mL × 60 microdrops = 48 microdrops (flow rate)

The formula for determining flow rate when a prescribed amount of medication per kilogram of body weight is ordered per minute is then:

$$\text{Flow Rate} = \frac{\text{Total Volume (mL)} \times \text{Drop Factor}}{\text{Total Amount of Medication}} \times \begin{array}{c}\text{Amount Medication}\\ \text{for Body Weight}\end{array}$$

EXAMPLE: Determine the flow rate for the following:

Prescribed medication: **0.5 mg per kg per minute**
Medication available: **2.0 g per 100 mL**
Weight of patient: **154 lb (70 kg)**
Drop factor: **60 microdrops per mL**

First, determine the mg for a person weighing 70 kg:

0.5 mg × 70 kg = 35 mg

Substituting in the formula:

$$\frac{\overset{3}{\cancel{100}} \text{ ml} \times \cancel{60} \text{ microdrops}}{\underset{20}{\cancel{2000}} \text{ mg}} \times 35 \text{ mg} = \begin{array}{l}105 \text{ microdrops/min}\\ \text{to deliver 0.5 mg/kg/min}\end{array}$$

---

*Note that in the second formula your answer will be in mL, which should be converted to drops per minute by multiplying by the drop factor.

The next formula shows how to determine medication received per minute.

$$\frac{\text{Total Amount Medication Prescribed}}{\text{Prescribed Time}} = \begin{array}{l}\text{Amount Medication}\\\text{Received per Minute}\end{array}$$

EXAMPLE: Determine the amount of Mezlin received per minute if the following order was written:

Prescribed medication:	**Mezlin 4 g**
Solution:	**100 mL**
Flow rate:	**34 drops per minute**
Length time to infuse:	**30 minutes**

Substituting in the formula:

$$\frac{4 \text{ g}}{30 \text{ min}} = 0.13 \text{ g per minute}$$

PRACTICE PROBLEMS

Determine the flow rate (drops per minute) and the amount of medication received per minute for the following problems:

1. Prescribed medication: Mefoxin 2 g per 100 mL solution (cefoxitin sodium)
   Specified time: 30 minutes
   Drop factor: 15 drops/mL

2. Prescribed medication: Ancef 1 g per 150 mL solution
   Specified time: 30 minutes
   Drop factor: 10 drops/mL

3. Prescribed medication: Gentamycin 80 mg per 100 mL
   Specified time: 45 minutes
   Drop factor: 60 microdrops/mL

Determine the flow rate for the following:

4. Prescribed medication: 5 mg Mefoxin (cefoxitin sodium) per minute
   Medication available: 0.5 g per 150 mL solution
   Drop factor: 10 drops/mL

5. Prescribed medication: Pipracel 50 mg per minute
   Medication available: 3 g per 100 mL
   Drop factor: 10 drops/mL

6. Prescribed medication: Terramycin (oxytetracycline HCl) 8 mg per minute
   Medication available: Terramycin 500 mg per 100 mL
   Drop factor: 10 drops/mL

Calculate: (1) the medication per kilogram body weight and (2) the flow rate for the following:

7. Prescribed medication: Achromycin 1 mg/kg/min
   Medication available: 250 mg per 100 mL
   Drop factor: 60 microdrops per 1 mL
   Weight of patient: 110 lb (50 kilograms)

8. Prescribed medication: Velosef 0.5 mg/kg/min
   Medication available: Velosef 1 g per 100 mL solution
   Drop factor: 10 guttae/mL
   Weight of patient: 154 lb (70 kg)

9. Prescribed medication: Pipracel 0.5 mg/kg/min
   Medication available: Pipracel 3 g per 100 mL
   Drop factor: 10 guttae/mL
   Weight of patient: 132 lb (60 kg)

Answers to Practice Problems

1. Flow rate is 50 drops per minute. 66 mg or 0.06 g Mefoxin per minute.
2. Flow rate is 50 drops per minute. 33 mg or 0.03 g Ancef per minute.
3. Flow rate is 133 microdrops per minute. 1.77 mg Gentamycin per minute.
4. Flow rate is 15 drops per minute.
5. Flow rate is 16.6 or 17 drops per minute.
6. Flow rate is 16 drops per minute.
7. 50 mg per minute for person who weighs 50 kilograms. Flow rate would be 1200 microdrops per minute.
8. 35 mg per minute for person who weighs 70 kg. Flow rate would be 35 drops per minute.
9. 30 mg per minute for person who weighs 60 kg. Flow rate would be 10 drops per minute.

ADDITIONAL PRACTICE PROBLEMS

Determine the flow rate and the amount of medication received per minute for the following:

1. Prescribed medication: Gentamycin 80 mg per 100 mL
   Specified time: 45 minutes
   Drop factor: 10 drops/mL

2. Prescribed medication: Penicillin G Sodium 50,000 units per 250 mL
   Specified time: 60 minutes
   Drop factor: 60 microdrops/mL

3. Prescribed medication: Velosef 2 g per 100 mL solution
   Specified time: 30 minutes
   Drop factor: 10 drops/mL

Determine the flow rate for the following:

4. Prescribed medication: Tetracycline 2 mg/min
   Medication available: Tetracycline 250 mg per 100 mL
   Drop factor: 10 drops/mL

5. Prescribed medication: Velosef 10 mg/min
   Medication available: 1 g per 100 mL
   Drop factor: 60 microdrops/mL

6. Prescribed medication: Pipracel 30 mg/min
   Medication available: Pipracel 2 g per 100 mL solution
   Drop factor: 10 drops/mL

Calculate the medication received per minute per kilogram body weight and the flow rate for the following:

7. Prescribed medication: Pipracel 15 mg/kg/wt/min
   Medication available: Pipracel 3 g per 100 mL
   Drop factor: 60 microdrops/mL
   Weight of patient: 176 lb (80 kg)

8. Prescribed medication: Mefoxin 1.5 mg/kg/min
   Medication available: Mefoxin 2 g per 100 mL
   Drop factor: 10 drops/mL
   Weight of patient: 121 lb (55 kg)

9. Prescribed medication: Gentamycin 0.02 mg/kg/min
   Medication available: Gentamycin 80 mg per 100 mL
   Drop factor: 60 microdrops/mL
   Weight of patient: 66 lb (30 kg)

Answers to Additional Practice Problems

1. Flow rate is 22 drops per minute. 1.77 mg Gentamycin per minute.
2. Flow rate is 250 microdrops per minute. 833 units Penicillin G per minute.
3. Flow rate is 33 drops per minute. 66 mg Velosef per minute.

4. Flow rate is 0.8 mL or 8 drops per minute.
5. Flow rate is 1 mL or 10 drops per minute.
6. Flow rate is 1.5 mL or 15 drops per minute.
7. 1200 mg per minute for person weighing 80 kg. Flow rate would be 2400 microdrops.
8. 82.5 mg per minute for person weighing 55 kg. Flow rate would be 41 or 42 drops per minute.
9. 0.6 mg Gentamycin per minute for person weighing 30 kg. Flow rate = 45 microguttae.

LESSON 14

Celsius and Fahrenheit Temperature Scales

Objectives

After completing this lesson, the student will be able to:

- State the formula for converting Fahrenheit to Celsius.

- State the formula for converting Celsius to Fahrenheit.

- Solve the problems at the end of this lesson with no more than one error.

The two scales used in measuring air, cooking, and body temperatures are Celsius (C)—also known as centigrade—and Fahrenheit (F). On the Celsius scale, the boiling point is 100° and the freezing point is 0°. On the Fahrenheit scale, the boiling point is 212° and the freezing point is 32°. One degree on the Fahrenheit scale equals $\frac{9}{5}$ of 1°C. One degree Celsius equals $\frac{5}{9}$ of 1°F.

Thermometers are available with either Celsius (centigrade) or Fahrenheit scales. Oral thermometers may have stubby, pear-shaped, or long tips. Those with stubby or pear-shaped tips are also used as rectal or axillary thermometers. Each division mark on the Fahrenheit scale represents 2°, whereas each division on the Celsius scale represents 1°.

The normal range of body temperature is from 36.5 to 37.5°C and from 97.6 to 99.4°F.

The formulas given below are used to convert from one scale to the other.

To Convert Fahrenheit to Celsius

$$(°F - 32) \times \frac{5}{9} = °C$$

EXAMPLE: Change 99°F to degrees Celsius.

Substitute in the formula just given:

$$(°F - 32) \times \frac{5}{9} = °C$$

$$(99° - 32) \times \frac{5}{9} = 67° \times \frac{5}{9} = 37.2°C$$

EXAMPLE: Change 102°F to degrees Celsius.

$$(102° - 32) \times \frac{5}{9} = 70° \times \frac{5}{9} = 38.8°C$$

To Convert Celsius to Fahrenheit

$$(°C \times \frac{9}{5}) + 32 = °F$$

EXAMPLE: Change 32°C to degrees Fahrenheit.

Substitute into the formula above:

$$\left(°C \times \frac{9}{5}\right) + 32 = °F$$

$$\left(32° \times \frac{9}{5}\right) + 32 = 57.6° + 32 = 89.6°F$$

EXAMPLE: Change 40°C to degrees Fahrenheit.

Substitute into formula as above:

$$\left(40° \times \frac{9}{5}\right) + 32 = 72° + 32 = 104°F$$

PRACTICE PROBLEMS

Convert the following degrees of temperature from the scale given to their equivalents in the other scale:

1. 98°F = _____   2. 104°F = _____

3. 45°C = _____   4. 100°F = _____

5. 100°C = _____   6. 95°F = _____

7. 35°C = _____   8. 99.6°F = _____

9. 30°C = _____   10. 101°F = _____

Answers to Practice Problems

1. 36.6°C	2. 40°C
3. 113°F	4. 37.7°C
5. 212°F	6. 35°C
7. 95°F	8. 37.5°C
9. 86°F	10. 38.3°C

If you made no more than one error, go on to Lesson 15. If not, review this lesson and try solving the problems again.

LESSON 15

Computing Dosages for Injection Using Tablets

Objective

After completing this lesson, the student will be able to:

* Solve the practice problems at the end of this lesson with no more than two errors.

The quantity of drug contained in tablets used in preparing dosages for hypodermic use is sometimes greater and sometimes less than the amount of drug ordered. This makes it necessary to use a fraction of a tablet or more than one tablet. However, since tablets are rather small and cannot be physically divided into accurate halves, thirds, etc (by breaking them), this fraction of a tablet is determined by dissolving the tablet or tablets in distilled water and then administering the amount of *solution* containing the correct dosage.

When the tablet on hand is smaller than the dose ordered, it is understood that two or more *whole* tablets will be required. The number of tablets needed should be ascertained first, and then *the total amount should be used as the dose on hand*. Remember, since these tablets cannot be broken, fractions must be rounded to the next *greater* whole number (ie, whole tablet).

The rule for determining the number of tablets needed takes the following form:

$$\frac{\text{Amount Ordered}}{\text{Amount on Hand}} = \text{Number of Tablets}$$

NOTE: Actually your answer will be the fractional dosage, but as emphasized above, this result is automatically rounded off to the next greater whole number: $\frac{1}{2}$ to 1, $1\frac{1}{5}$ to 2, $2\frac{3}{4}$ to 3, etc.

EXAMPLE: Give morphine grain $\frac{1}{6}$ from tablets grain $\frac{1}{8}$.

It is evident that $\frac{1}{6}$ is larger than $\frac{1}{8}$ and that it will be necessary to determine the number of tablets needed. Using the formula above, we have:

$$\frac{\frac{1}{6}}{\frac{1}{8}} = \frac{1}{6} \times \frac{8}{1} = \frac{8}{6} = 1\frac{1}{3} \text{ or (rounding off) 2 tablets}$$

In working out a complete tablet problem (see below), the drug on hand would thus be 2 tablets grain $\frac{1}{8}$ each for a total of grain $\frac{1}{4}$.

Dosage problems using tablets are worked by the same formulas as given in Lesson 7 on parenteral dosages, and you can use either of the formulas given there (repeated below) to solve problems. Since this medication is not in solution, your calculations will be simplified if you take the dilution to be 1 cc.

Formula 1

Drug on Hand : Dilution (1 cc) :: Drug Ordered : x (Amount to Administer)

Formula 2 (Shortened Version of Formula 1)

$$\frac{\text{Dose Ordered}}{\text{Drug on Hand}} \times 1 \text{ cc} = \text{Amount to Administer}$$

EXAMPLE: Give morphine grain $\frac{1}{6}$ from tablets grain $\frac{1}{8}$.

From the result of the previous example above, we know that drug on hand is 2 tablets or grain $\frac{1}{4}$. Substitute in Formula 2 and solve:

$$\frac{\text{Dose Ordered}}{\text{Drug on Hand}} \times 1 \text{ cc} = \text{Amount to Administer}$$

$$\frac{\text{grain } \frac{1}{6}}{\text{grain } \frac{1}{4}} \times 1 \text{ cc} = \frac{1}{\underset{3}{6}} \times \frac{\overset{2}{4}}{1} \times 1 \text{ cc} = \frac{2}{3} \text{ cc or 11 minims}$$

Answer: Dissolve 2 tablets of morphine grain $\frac{1}{8}$ each in 1 cc (16 minims) sterile water, discard 5 minims and administer 11 minims = grain $\frac{1}{6}$.

Do not change from one system to another (Apothecaries' to Metric and vice versa) unless necessary. If the dosage is ordered in Metric units, ie, grams or milligrams, do not convert to grains, but solve as given.

EXAMPLE: Give 0.01 g of morphine from 0.016-g tablets.

Substituting in Formula 2, you would have the following:

$$\frac{0.01}{0.016} \times 1 \text{ cc} = \frac{1}{\cancel{100}} \times \frac{\overset{10}{\cancel{1000}}}{16} \times 1 \text{ cc}$$

$$= \frac{10}{16} = 0.62 \text{ or (rounding off the decimal fraction)}$$
$$0.6 \text{ cc or 10 minims}$$

Answer: Dissolve 1 tablet of 0.016 g morphine in 1 cc (= 16 minims) of distilled water, discard 6 minims, and give 10 minims, which contain 0.01 g morphine.

NOTE: Since it is easier to work with whole numbers, the problem above would be simplified if the fractional grams were changed to milligrams by mentally moving the decimal point three places to the right:

$$\frac{0.01}{0.0016} \text{ to } \frac{10}{16}$$

NOTE: If the drug ordered and the drug on hand are not in the same system or same units, you should convert all the quantities to one system, choosing the one that will make your calculations easier.

NOTE: If answer in minims is larger than dilution chosen when using tablets, you have made an error either in calculation or have not used enough tablets.

In the following problem we make the error of not using enough tablets.

EXAMPLE: Give morphine grain $\frac{1}{6}$ from tablets grain $\frac{1}{8}$.

Substitute these values into Formula 2:

$$\frac{\frac{1}{6}}{\frac{1}{8}} \times 1 \text{ cc} = \frac{1}{\overset{}{\underset{3}{6}}} \times \frac{\overset{4}{\cancel{8}}}{1} \times 1 \text{ cc} = \frac{4}{3} \text{ or } 1\frac{1}{3} \text{ cc}$$

If you will study this problem closely, you will see that something is wrong. You have put a tablet in a given amount of solution (1 cc), but somehow you miraculously come up with an extra $\frac{1}{3}$ cc. The error is that you cannot get $\frac{1}{6}$ from $\frac{1}{8}$; therefore, 2 tablets of grain $\frac{1}{8}$ will have to be used, which will make the dose on hand $\frac{2}{8}$ or grain $\frac{1}{4}$. The correct working out of the problem is as follows:

$$\frac{\frac{1}{6}}{\frac{1}{4}} \times 1 \text{ cc} = \frac{1}{\overset{}{\underset{3}{6}}} \times \frac{\overset{2}{\cancel{4}}}{1} \times 1 \text{ cc} = \frac{2}{3} \text{ cc or 10 minims}$$

Thus, dissolve 2 tablets of morphine grain $\frac{1}{8}$ each in 1 cc distilled water, discard 6 minims, and give 10 minims.

PRACTICE PROBLEMS

The following problems ask you to prepare injections using tablets. State your answers in minims.

Physician's Orders	Label on Bottle
1. Scopolamine grain $\frac{1}{300}$ (H) @ 8 AM	Scopolamine hydrobromide 0.6-mg tablets
2. Dilaudid grain $\frac{1}{32}$ (H) stat	Hydromorphone HCl (Dilaudid) 2.5-mg tab
3. Apomorphine grain $\frac{1}{24}$ (H) stat	Apomorphine HCl 5-mg tab
4. Atropine grain $\frac{1}{120}$ (H) @ 7:30 AM	Atropine sulfate 0.4-mg tab
5. Pantopon grain $\frac{1}{3}$ IM q 4 hr prn for pain	Omnopon (Pantopon) 10-mg tab
6. Codeine grain ss (H) q 4 hr prn for pain	Codeine phosphate 60-mg tab
7. Morphine grain $\frac{1}{4}$ q 4 hr prn for pain	Morphine sulfate 10-mg tab
8. Strychnine sulfate grain $\frac{1}{50}$ (H) tid	Strychnine sulfate 2-mg tab
9. Dilaudid 0.0032 g q 4 hr prn for pain	Hydromorphone HCl (Dilaudid) 2.5-mg tab
10. Morphine grain $\frac{1}{6}$ (H) q 3-4 hr prn for pain	Morphine sulfate 0.008 g tab
11. Digitoxin grain $\frac{1}{100}$ (H) stat	Digitoxin grain $\frac{1}{120}$ tab

12. Atropine grain $\frac{1}{100}$ (H) @ 8 AM   Atropine sulfate 0.6-mg tab

13. Scopolamine 0.4 mg (H) @
    9 AM

    Scopolamine hydrobromide
    0.0004-g tab

14. Pantopon 0.02 g IM q 4
    hr prn for pain

    Omnopon (Pantopon)
    grain $\frac{1}{6}$ (10-mg) tab

15. Apomorphine grain $\frac{1}{48}$ (H) stat   Apomorphine HCl 0.005 g
    tab

Answers to Practice Problems

1. 5 minims. [Dissolve 1 tab scopolamine 0.6 mg in 1 mL water, discard 11 minims, and give 5 minims, which equal grain $\frac{1}{300}$.]
2. 12 minims. [Dissolve 1 tab hydromorphone 2.5 mg in 1 mL water, discard 4 minims, and give 12 minims, which equal grain $\frac{1}{32}$.]
3. 8 minims. [Dissolve 1 tab 5 mg in 1 mL water, discard 8 minims, and give 8 minims, which equal grain $\frac{1}{24}$.]
4. 10 minims. [0.4 mg = grain $\frac{1}{150}$. So 2 tablets are needed. Drug on hand is $\frac{1}{150} + \frac{1}{150} = \frac{2}{150}$ or $\frac{1}{75}$. Substituting in formula,

$$\frac{\frac{1}{75}}{\frac{1}{120}} \times 1\text{ mL} = \frac{1}{\overset{}{\underset{8}{\cancel{120}}}} \times \frac{\overset{5}{\cancel{75}}}{1} \times 1\text{ mL} = \frac{5}{8}\text{ mL or 10 minims.}$$]

5. 16 minims. [10 mg = grain $\frac{1}{6}$. Then 2 tab grain $\frac{1}{6}$ = grain $\frac{1}{3}$. So dissolve 2 tab 10 mg of omnopon in 1 mL of sterile water.]
6. 8 minims.
7. 12 minims. [Did you forget to use 2 tablets?]
8. 9 minims.
9. 10 minims.
10. 10 minims. [0.008 g = grain $\frac{1}{8}$, so 2 tablets are needed.]
11. 10 minims.
12. 16 minims. [Since 0.6 mg = grain $\frac{1}{100}$, dissolve 1 tab 0.6 mg atropine in 1 mL sterile water and give. Or, you could use 0.5 cc or any amount that dissolved the tablet well.]
13. 16 minims. [Since 0.0004 g = 0.4 mg, dissolve 1 tab 0.4 mg Scopolamine in 1 mL sterile water and give.]

14. 16 minims. [0.02 g = 20 mg. Dissolve 2 tab grain $\frac{1}{6}$ (10 mg) in 1 mL sterile water and give.]
15. 4 minims. [0.005 g = 5 mg = grain $\frac{1}{12}$. Dissolve 1 tablet apomorphine in 1 mL sterile water, discard 12 minims, and give 4 minims.]

If you made no more than two errors, go on to Lesson 16. If not, review the lesson and try to solve the problems again.

LESSON 16

Measuring Minims

Objectives

After completing this lesson, without referring to a book, the student will be able to:

- State how minims and fractions of minims are measured.

- Solve the practice problems at the end of this lesson with no more than 1 error.

A minim glass or minim pipette should be used to measure minims. Minim glasses are marked off in 5's or multiples of 5; therefore, pour the next highest multiple of 5 above the required dosage, dilute five times, and give of the dilution as many minims as five times the dose ordered.

EXAMPLE: Give *m* viii of tincture of hyoscyamus.

First, pour 10 minims of the tincture and then dilute five times by adding 40 minims of water. You now have the following equivalents:

1 minim = 5 minims
10 minims of drug = 50 minims of solution
8 minims of drug = 40 minims of solution

To measure a fraction of a minim, do the following:

1. Pour 5 minims.
2. Dilute as many times as five times the denominator of dose wanted.
3. Take as many minims of dilution as five times the numerator of dose wanted.

EXAMPLE: Measure _m_ ss ($\frac{1}{2}$) of a drug.

Proceed as follows:

1. Pour 5 minims.
2. Dilute 10 times, or add 45 minims of water.
3. Give 5 minims.

NOTE: If you dilute correctly in measuring fractions of a minim, the amount given will always be 5 minims, if numerator is one.

PRACTICE PROBLEMS

In the following problems state your answer for the amounts to pour, give, and administer.

1. Measure *m* ix of hydrochloric acid.

2. Measure *m* xiii of a drug.

3. Measure *m* xx of a drug.

4. Measure *m* $\frac{1}{4}$ of a drug.

5. Measure *m* $\frac{1}{5}$ of a drug.

Answers to Practice Problems

1. Pour *m* x, add *m* xl (40) of water, and administer *m* xlv (45) of solution. This will equal *m* ix of the drug.
2. Pour *m* xv, add *m* lx (60) of water, and give *m* lxv (65) for a dose of *m* xiii of drug.
3. Pour *m* xx, add *m* lxxx of water, and give to patient. Or, pour the *m* xx and put in $\frac{1}{2}$ to $\frac{1}{4}$ glass of water and give.
4. Pour *m* v, dilute 20 times (five times the denominator: $5 \times 4 = 20$) by adding 95 minims of water ($100 - 5$), and give *m* v for the *m* $\frac{1}{4}$ dose.
5. Pour *m* v, dilute 25 times (5×5) by adding 120 minims of water ($125 - 5$), and give *m* v.

If you made no more than one error, go on to Lesson 17. If not, review the lesson and try to solve the problems again.

LESSON 17

Preparing Solutions from Pure Drugs

Objectives

After completing this lesson, and without referring to a book, the student will be able to:

- Solve ten problems to determine the amount of solute needed with no more than one error.
- Solve ten problems to determine the amount of solvent needed with no more than one error.
- Solve ten problems to determine the percentage or ratio strength of a solution with no more than one error.

Today nursing students are required to make very few solutions since most of them are made by the pharmacist. Occasionally, however, the nurse does have to make up solutions for enemas, douches, or irrigations, and you must therefore develop the ability to make solutions accurately and quickly.

A *solution* is a clear, homogeneous mixture with a tendency to settle out on standing. The parts of a solution are the *solvent* and the *solute*. The solvent is the liquid in which the solute, ie, the drug, is dissolved.

Solution strengths are expressed in percent or as a ratio; eg, 10% dextrose in water means that there are 10 parts of dextrose to 100 parts of water or that there are 10 g of dextrose per 100 mL of water or that the ratio strength is 10 : 100 or 1 : 10.

SOLVING SOLUTION PROBLEMS

Solution problems are calculated more accurately and more easily if amounts are converted to the Metric system, ie, grains to grams and ounces, pints and quarts to milliliters or cubic centimeters. Since solution problems are calculated by using the proportion formula, units must not only be in the same system, but must also be in equal terms, ie, the proportion must be balanced:

cc : g :: cc : g

and not

cc : g :: g : cc

EXAMPLE: What is the ratio strength of a solution which contains grain xv of sodium chloride to 1 qt of water?

Grains and quarts are both in the Apothecaries' system, but are not equal terms. Equal terms are grams and cubic centimeters (milliliters). Grains and minims are also equal terms, but they are not used in calculating solution problems since large amounts such as quarts and pints are involved. The quart should be changed to milliliters and the grains to grams for both units to be in the same system and in equal terms:

1 qt = 1000 mL *and* grain xv = 1 g

The ratio strength of a solution which has grain xv sodium chloride (1 g) per quart (1000 mL) of water would be a 1 : 1000 solution, or a solution with 1 part of sodium chloride to 1000 parts of water.

Formulas for Solution Problems

All solution problems can be worked by using the formulas given below with the one exception that is given later.

$$
\text{Drug : Water :: Percent : 100}
$$
$$
or
$$
$$
\frac{\text{Desired Strength}}{\text{Available Strength}} = \frac{\text{Amount to Use}}{\text{Amount to Make}}
$$

The strength of a pure drug is 100%. The above proportion formula is used when solutions are made from pure drugs.

EXAMPLE: Make 1 qt of a 5% solution of sodium bicarbonate.

The amount of water (solvent) and the percent solution desired are given. Since no other percent or ratio is given, you know that your available drug is pure or 100%. Solve for the amount of sodium bicarbonate, which is the unknown, by substituting in the proportion formula after converting the quart to cubic centimeters:

Drug : Water :: Percent : 100

x g : 1000 cc :: 5% : 100%

NOTE: x in this case is in grams since the soda is a powder. The answer will also be in grams, rather than cubic centimeters.

Multiply extremes and means and solve for x:

100 x = 5000

x = 50 g

Answer: Weigh out 50 g of soda into a quart container and add 950 cc water, which will give 1000 cc of a 5% solution of soda.

NOTE: Although the soda in the above example was weighed out in grams, most solutions that a nurse would be required to make are made by measuring the amount of drug in a medicine glass or graduated measuring cup since 1 cc weighs approximately 1 g and the two are essentially equal. If the drug is potent, it should be weighed on a gram scale.

FINDING THE PERCENTAGE STRENGTH OF A SOLUTION

EXAMPLE: If a solution contains 5 g of drug to 1000 cc of water, what percent is the solution?

In this problem you have the amount of drug and the amount of water given. The percentage strength is the unknown. Substitute the known values into the proportion formula:

5 g : 1000 cc :: x : 100%

1000 x = 500

x = 0.5%

NOTE: Since the ratio is set up as percent to 100, the answer is already in percent and does not have to be changed.

EXAMPLE: If a solution has grain xxx of drug to 1 qt of water, what percent is the solution?

Remember, the terms of the proportion must be in the same system as well as in equal or equivalent terms, so the grains and the quart must be converted: grain xxx = 2 g and 1 qt = 1000 cc. Substituting in the formula:

$$2 \text{ g} : 1000 \text{ cc} :: x : 100\%$$

$$1000 \, x = 200$$

$$x = 0.2\%$$

DETERMINING THE AMOUNT OF WATER NEEDED

EXAMPLE: How much water is needed to make a 2% solution from 0.2 g of potassium permanganate?

Substituting in the formula:

$$0.2 \text{ g} : x \text{ mL} :: 2\% : 100\%$$

$$2x = 20$$

$$x = 10 \text{ mL}$$

EXAMPLE: How much water is needed to make a 1% salt solution using 1 oz of sodium chloride?

Converting to the same system and to equivalent terms: 1 oz = 30 cc or 30 g. Then substituting in the formula:

$$30 \text{ g} : x \text{ cc} :: 1\% : 100\%$$

$$x = 3000 \text{ cc}$$

Answer: Add 2970 cc to 30 g of salt to make a 1% solution.

PRACTICE PROBLEMS

Indicate how much of the pure drug is needed to make up the amount of solution called for.

Amount of Solute

1. Make 1 gallon of a 5% solution of magnesium sulfate for hot packs.

2. Make 1 pint of $\frac{1}{2}$% Lysol solution.

3. Make 3 liters of 1% solution of boric acid.

4. Make 1 liter of a 2% solution of potassium permanganate.

5. Make 1 gallon of a 0.5% solution.

6. Make 1 quart of a 1% solution.

7. Make 2 gallons of a 10% solution.

8. Make a half pint of a 1% solution of argyrol.

9. Make 2 ounces of a $\frac{1}{4}$% solution of merbromin (Mercurochrome).

10. Make 1 quart of 1% solution of sodium chloride.

Percentage or Ratio Strength

11. What percent is a solution of 12 g of drug per gallon of water?

12. What percent is a solution of grain xxx of drug in 2000 cc of water?

13. What percent is a solution of 500 mg of drug per ounce of solvent?

14. What percent is a solution which has 0.5 g of drug per 100 cc water?

15. What percent is a solution which has 20 cc of pure drug per 1000 cc water?

16. What percent is a solution of grain x of drug per ounce of water?

17. What is the ratio strength of a solution which has 1 g of drug per pint of water?

18. What is the ratio strength of a solution with 1 g of drug in 2 cc water?

19. What is the strength of a solution which has 5 g of drug dissolved in a gallon of water?

20. What is the strength of a solution which has 1 oz of pure drug in a quart of water?

Amount of Solvent

21. How much water is needed to make a 4% solution using 15 cc Lysol?

22. How much water is needed to make a 0.9% sodium chloride solution using 45 g of salt?

23. How much 5% solution can be made from a grain xv tablet?

24. How much 10% solution can be made from 1 oz of salt?

25. How much water is needed to make a $\frac{1}{2}$% solution using 1 g boric acid crystals?

26. How much 1% solution can be made from a 1-g tablet?

27. How much 5% solution can be made from 3 t (teaspoonsful) of salt?

28. How much $\frac{1}{2}$% solution can be made from a potassium permanganate tablet of 0.3 g?

29. How much water is needed to make a $\frac{1}{4}$% solution using a grain v tablet?

30. How much water is needed to make a 20% solution of mercuric chloride using a 0.5-g tablet?

Answers to Practice Problems

1. 200 g. [Measure 200 g (200 cc magnesium sulfate crystals) in a gallon container, add 3800 cc water to make 1 gal (4000 cc) of a 5% solution.]
2. 2.5 cc (Lysol is a liquid). [Add 497.5 cc water to make 1 pt of $\frac{1}{2}$% sol.]
3. 30 g or cc
4. 20 g or cc
5. 20 g or cc
6. 10 g
7. 800 g
8. 2.5 g or cc
9. 0.15 g
10. 10 g or cc
11. 0.3%. [Remember, your answer is already a percent, not a decimal fraction.]
12. 0.1%. [You didn't forget to convert grains to grams, did you? Metric system for solutions!]
13. 1.6%. [Milligrams are a Metric unit but are not equivalent with cubic centimeters. Only grams and cubic centimeters are.]
14. $\frac{1}{2}$%
15. 2%
16. 2%
17. 1 : 500
18. 1 : 2
19. $\frac{1}{8}$%
20. 3%
21. 375 cc
22. 5000 cc. [Did you forget to move your decimal point when dividing by 0.9?]
23. 20 cc. [If you did not convert the grain xv to grams, your answer would be 300 minims. When preparing solutions, however, the Metric system should be used.]
24. 300 cc
25. 200 cc. [Don't forget to invert the divisor.]
26. 100 cc
27. 240 cc. [Keep reviewing those tables!]
28. 60 cc
29. 120 cc
30. 2.5 cc

If you made no more than one error in each section, go on to Lesson 18. If not, review the lesson and try to solve the problems again.

LESSON 18

Preparing a Given Amount of a Weaker Solution from a Stronger Solution

Objectives

After completing this lesson, the student will be able to:

- Calculate solution problems when the solution on hand is not a pure drug and the percentage strength is given.

- Solve solution problems when only the ratio strength of the desired solution is given.

- Solve solution problems when two ratio strengths are given.

- Solve solution problems when the strength of one solution is given as a percent and one as a ratio.

- Explain why the ratio strength can be substituted for the "Percent : 100" term in the solution formula.

- Solve the practice problems at the end of this lesson with no more than two errors.

If the drug available is not a pure drug (100%), and the percent of the solution is given, the desired strength is substitute for the 100% in the formula given in Lesson 17.

MAKING SOLUTIONS WHEN TWO PERCENTAGES ARE KNOWN

For this type of problem the formula given in the previous lesson, ie, Drug : Water :: Percent : 100, may be changed to one of the following formulas:

Drug : Water :: Percent Solution Wanted : Solution on Hand

or

$$\frac{\text{Desired Strength}}{\text{Available Strength}} = \frac{\text{Amount to Use}}{\text{Amount to Make}}$$

EXAMPLE: Make 1 pt of a 1% solution from a 10% stock solution.

Substitute the known values into the proportion formula above:

Drug : Water :: Percent Solution Wanted : Solution on Hand

x cc : 500 cc :: 1% : 10%

$10x = 500$

$x = 50$ cc

NOTE: The unknown, x, will be in cubic centimeters or milliliters since you are dealing with solutions.

Answer: Pour out 50 cc of the 10% solution of Lysol solution into a pint container and add enough water (450 cc) to make 1 pt (500 cc). This will make 1 pt of a 1% solution of Lysol.

Or you can proceed as follows using the equation given above:

$$\frac{\text{Desired Strength}}{\text{Available Strength}} = \frac{\text{Amount to Use}}{\text{Amount to Make}}$$

$$\frac{1\%}{10\%} = \frac{x \text{ cc}}{500 \text{ cc}}$$

$10x = 500$

$x = 50$ cc

EXAMPLE: Make 2 qt of a $\frac{1}{2}$% solution from a 5% solution.

Substitute in the formula:

$$x \text{ cc} : 2000 \text{ cc} :: \frac{1}{2}\% : 5\%$$

$$5x = 1000$$

$$x = 200 \text{ cc}$$

Answer: Measure 200 cc from the 5% stock solution and add 1800 cc of water to make 2 qt of a $\frac{1}{2}\%$ solution.

MAKING WEAKER SOLUTIONS WHEN A RATIO STRENGTH IS GIVEN

In problems such as these, the solution ratio desired is substituted for both the percent term and the 100(%) in the proportion formula previously given (Drug : Water :: Percent : 100), and *only* the desired ratio strength is used (since it is, of course, a ratio itself). Thus, the formula takes the following form:

> Drug : Water :: Ratio Strength of Solution Desired

EXAMPLE: Make a gallon of a 1 : 4000 solution of boric acid.

To find your answer substitute the known values in the formula given above and solve:

Drug : Water :: Ratio Strength Desired

$$x \text{ g} : 4000 \text{ cc} :: 1 : 4000$$

$$4000x = 4000$$

$$x = 1 \text{ g}$$

Answer: Measure 1 g or 1 cc boric acid crystals into a gallon container and add enough water (3999 cc) to make a gallon of 1 : 4000 solution.

If you had converted the ratio 1 : 4000 to a percent, you would have gotten $\frac{1}{40}\%$. Then, $\frac{1}{40} : 100$ or $\frac{1}{40} \div 100 = \frac{1}{4000}$ or 1 : 4000; therefore, by substituting the ratio in the formula, you not only save time, but also eliminate the chance of errors.

MAKING WEAKER SOLUTIONS WHEN TWO RATIO STRENGTHS ARE GIVEN

When you are given the two ratio strengths from which to make a solution, you should convert the ratios to fractions and use the following variation of the proportional formula:

Drug : Water :: Desired Ratio : Available Ratio
(as a fraction)   (as a fraction)

EXAMPLE: Make 1 qt of a 1 : 1000 solution from a 1 : 200 solution.

Substitute the known values in the proportion as given above and solve the resulting equation after multiplying the means and extremes:

Drug : Water :: Desired Ratio : Available Ratio

$$x \text{ cc} : 1000 :: \frac{1}{1000} : \frac{1}{200}$$

$$\frac{1}{200} x = \frac{\frac{1}{1000}}{\frac{1000}{1}}$$

$$x = \frac{200}{1} = 200 \text{ cc}$$

Answer: Measure 200 cc of the 1 : 200 solution in a quart container and add 800 cc of water, which gives 1000 cc of a 1 : 1000 solution.

MAKING SOLUTIONS WHEN A RATIO AND A PERCENT ARE GIVEN

In this type problem, the percent should be converted to a fraction, since this is easier than converting the ratio to a percent.

EXAMPLE: Make 1 gal of a 1 : 5000 solution from a $\frac{1}{2}$% solution.

Convert the $\frac{1}{2}$% to a fraction:

$$\tfrac{1}{2}\% = \frac{1}{2} \div 100 = \frac{1}{2} \times \frac{1}{100} = \frac{1}{200}$$

Then, writing the $1:5000$ as a fraction, substitute the values in the formula:

Drug : Water :: Desired Strength : Available Strength

$$x \text{ cc} : 4000 \text{ cc} :: \frac{1}{5000} : \frac{1}{200}$$

$$\frac{1}{200}x = \frac{4000}{5000}$$

$$x = \frac{\overset{4}{\cancel{4000}}}{\underset{5}{\cancel{5000}}} \times \frac{\overset{40}{\cancel{200}}}{1} = 160 \text{ cc}$$

Answer: Measure 160 cc of the $\frac{1}{2}$% solution into a gallon container and add 3840 cc of water to make 1 gal of a $1:5000$ solution.

EXAMPLE: Make 1 qt of a $\frac{1}{4}$% solution from a $1:100$ solution.

Substitute in the formula:

$$x \text{ cc} : 1000 \text{ cc} :: \frac{1}{400} : \frac{1}{100}$$

$$\frac{1}{100}x = \frac{1000}{400}$$

$$x = \frac{\overset{10}{\cancel{1000}}}{\underset{4}{\cancel{400}}} \times \frac{\overset{25}{\cancel{100}}}{1} = 250 \text{ cc}$$

In this problem, your calculation would be simplified if the $1:100$ were converted to percent (1%). Therefore, when a ratio and a percent are given, convert to whichever is easier for you to use. Substituting in the formula after converting $1:100$ to 1%, one has:

$$x \text{ cc} : 1000 \text{ cc} :: \frac{1}{4}\% : 1\%$$

$$x = 250 \text{ cc}$$

Answer: Measure 250 cc of the $1:100$ solution add enough water (750 cc) to make 1 qt of a $\frac{1}{4}$% solution.

PRACTICE PROBLEMS

Indicate how much of the stock solution (stronger solution) is needed to make up the weaker solutions.

1. Make 2 quarts of a $\frac{1}{2}$% solution from a 5% solution.

2. Make 1 liter of a 1 : 4000 solution from a 1 : 1000 solution.

3. Make 1 gallon of a 1 : 4000 solution from a 1% solution.

4. Make 4 liters of a 1 : 20 solution from a 20% solution.

5. Make 3 quarts of a 2% solution from a 1 : 3 stock solution.

6. Make 1 pint of a $\frac{1}{4}$% solution from a 2% solution.

7. Make 3 liters of a 1 : 5000 bichloride of mercury solution from a 1 : 500 solution.

8. Make $\frac{1}{2}$ gallon of sodium chloride 1% solution from a 5% solution.

9. Prepare 2 liters of a 1 : 1000 bichloride of mercury solution from a $\frac{1}{2}$% stock solution.

10. Prepare 1 gallon of a 1 : 2000 solution from a 1 : 500 solution.

11. Prepare 1 liter of a 1% solution of soda bicarbonate.

12. Prepare 1 gallon of a 1 : 4000 solution of potassium permanganate.

13. Prepare 1 pint of a 1 : 500 solution of Lysol.

14. Prepare 2 liters of a 1 : 2000 solution of sodium chloride.

15. Prepare 1 gallon of a 1 : 4000 solution from a $\frac{1}{4}$% solution.

Answers to Practice Problems

The answers will be in cc's since you are making a weaker solution from a stronger solution.

1. 200 cc
2. 250 cc
3. 100 cc
4. 40 cc
5. 20 cc
6. 62.5 cc
7. 300 cc
8. 400 cc
9. 400 cc
10. 1000 cc
11. 10 g or cc
12. 1 cc or 1 g
13. 1 cc
14. 1 g or 1 cc
15. 400 cc

If you made no more than two errors, go on to Lesson 19. If not, review the lesson and try to solve the problems again.

LESSON 19

Making Solutions from Tablets

Objectives

After completing this lesson, and without referring to a book, the student will be able to:

- Describe the two steps used to solve problems to prepare solutions from tablets.

- State the formula for determining the number of tablets needed to prepare solutions.

- Solve solution problems in which tablets are utilized.

- Solve problems in preparing solutions from pure drugs.

- Solve problems in making a given quantity of a weaker solution from a stronger solution.

- Solve the practice problems at the end of this lesson with no more than two errors.

There are two steps in preparing solutions using tablets. First, the amount of drug needed will have to be determined, and then the number of tablets.

The formula for determining the number of tablets follows:

$$\frac{\text{Amount of Drug Wanted}}{\text{Drug on Hand}} = \text{Number of Tablets Needed}$$

NOTE: In preparing solutions, the number of tablets required is rounded off to the nearest whole number. Doing so will, of course, actually result in a slightly different ratio strength of the solution being prepared, but this difference is not likely to be significant.

EXAMPLE: Make $\frac{1}{2}$ gallon of a $1:4000$ solution of potassium permanganate using tablets grain v each.

The amount of drug needed to make 2000 cc of a $1:4000$ solution is not known. The tablets on hand are grain v. Substitute these values in the proportion formula and solve the resulting equation:

Drug : Water :: Percent : 100

x g : 2000 cc :: 1 : 4000

$4000x = 2000$

$$x = \frac{1}{2} \text{ or } 0.5 \text{ g}$$

Since the available tablets are labeled in grains, the grains must be converted to grams:

$$\text{grain v} = \frac{5 \text{ grain}}{15 \text{ grain}} = \frac{1}{3} \text{ or } 0.3 \text{ g}$$

$$x = \frac{1}{3} \text{ or } 0.3 \text{ g (rounded off to the nearest tenth of a gram)}$$

To determine the number of 5-grain (0.3-g) tablets, substitute in the formula for determining the number of tablets:

$$\frac{0.5}{0.3} = \frac{5}{10} \div \frac{3}{10} = \frac{5}{\cancel{10}} \times \frac{\cancel{10}}{3} = \frac{5}{3} = 1\frac{2}{3} \text{ or 2 tablets}$$

or

$$0.3 \overline{)0.5} \quad \underset{\cup \quad \cup}{\overset{1.6 \text{ tablets}}{}}$$

Answer: Place 2 tablets of potassium permanganate grain v each in 2000 cc water to make $\frac{1}{2}$ gallon of a 1 : 4000 solution.

EXAMPLE: Make a gallon of a 2% soda bicarbonate solution using grain x tablets.

Remembering that the soda is pure drug (100%) since it is a powder, substitute in formula:

$$x \text{ g} : 4000 \text{ cc} :: 2\% : 100\%$$

$$100x = 8000$$

$$x = 80 \text{ g}$$

Thus, 80 g of soda are needed to make the solution, but the number of tablets is unknown; therefore, if 1 tablet equals grain x, or 0.66 g, then

$$\begin{array}{r} 121.2 = 121 \text{ tablets} \\ 0.66\overline{)80.00} \end{array}$$

Answer: Place 121 tablets of soda grain x each in a gallon container and add 4000 cc of water to make a 2% solution of soda bicarbonate.

EXAMPLE: Prepare 2 liters of a 1 : 1000 bichloride of mercury solution using 0.5 g tablets.

Substitute in the formula:

$$x \text{ g} : 2000 \text{ cc} :: 1 : 1000$$

$$1000x = 2000$$

$$x = 2 \text{ g}$$

The amount of bichloride needed is 2 g. Since the tablets are labeled in grams, divide 2 g by 0.5 g, which equals 4 tablets.

PRACTICE PROBLEMS

Answer the following problems by indicating the solution strength (%) or by giving the amount of solution (in cc's) or the total weight (in mg's) and number of tablets to make the solutions required.

1. Prepare 1 gallon of normal saline (0.9%) solution using common table salt. How would you measure the amount of salt, since there are no scales for measuring grams?

2. Make 1 quart of a $\frac{1}{5}$% solution from a 2% solution.

3. Prepare 1 quart of a 1 : 2000 potassium permangante solution using grain iii tablets.

4. How much water will you need to make a $\frac{1}{2}$% solution using 2 g of sodium chloride?

5. Make 2 liters of a $\frac{1}{2}$% solution from a 5% solution.

6. Make 1 quart of a 10% magnesium sulfate solution.

7. Make 1 liter of a 1 : 1000 solution of bichloride.

8. Make 1 quart of a solution containing 4% glucose and 2% soda bicarbonate.

9. What is the percentage strength of a solution that contains 2 g of drug per 50 cc water?

10. How much water is needed to make a $\frac{1}{10}$% solution from 1 g of boric acid crystals?

11. If 0.5 g of salt is placed in 1 gallon of water, what is the strength of this solution?

12. With 7 tablets grain v of potassium permanganate make a saturated solution (7%). Read this problem carefully and compare with Problem 13 before solving.

13. Make 3 liters of a 1 : 3000 solution of bichloride using tablets grain viiss each.

14. Calculate the amount of acriflavine needed to make 1 pint of a 1 : 2000 solution.

15. Prepare 1 quart of a 1 : 2000 solution from a 1 : 100 solution.

16. Prepare 1.5 liters of a 1 : 1500 solution from a 1% solution.

17. What is the percentage strength of a solution which has grain xv of sodium chloride per liter?

18. Prepare 250 ml of a 1 : 5 solution from 5-g tablets.

19. A solution labeled 50% means that there is (are) _____ part(s) of drug to _____ part(s) of water. Written as a ratio, this would be _____ .

Answers to Practice Problems

1. 36 g. [Measure 36 cc in graduate or measuring cup, place in a gallon container, and add water to make 4000 cc.]
2. 100 cc. [Measure 100 cc of the 2% solution, pour into a quart container, and add 900 cc water to make a quart of $\frac{1}{5}$% solution.]
3. 0.5 g, 3 tablets
4. 400 cc
5. 200 cc
6. 100 g or cc
7. 1 g
8. 40 g glucose and 20 g soda. [Solve for glucose and then soda. Measure 40 cc glucose and 20 cc soda, place in a quart container, and add enough water (940 cc) to make 1000 cc.]
9. 4%
10. 1000 cc
11. $\frac{1}{80}$%
12. 33 cc. [In this problem you are solving for the amount of water to be added to 7 tablets, grain v each (35 grains or 2.3 g).]
13. 1 g, 2 tablets
14. 0.25 g

15. 50 cc
16. 100 cc
17. 0.1%
18. 50 g, 10 tablets
19. 1, 2, 1 : 2 solution

If you made no more than two errors, go on to Lesson 20. If not, review the lesson and try to solve the problems again.

LESSON 20

Preparing a Weaker Solution from a Given Amount of a Stronger Solution

Objectives

After completing this lesson, the student will be able to:

- Understand the difference between preparing weaker solutions from a given amount of a stronger solution and making a given quantity of a weaker solution from a stronger solution.

- State the formula for preparing weaker solutions from a given amount of a stronger solution without referring to the text.

- Solve problems for preparing weaker solutions from a given amount of a stronger solution.

- Solve the practice problems at the end of this lesson with no more than one error.

The one exception mentioned in Lesson 17 concerning formulas for making solutions is the one that will be used to determine the quantity of a weaker solution that may be made from a *given amount* of a stronger solution. In this type problem two percentages, two ratios, or a percentage and a ratio and one dilution are given. One diluent is to be found. You have a *given* quantity of a stronger solution to which you will add an *unknown* amount of water to make a weaker solution. *One formula used to make a weaker solution from a given amount of a stronger solution* is the following:

Greater : Lesser :: Greater : Lesser
Percent   Percent   Quantity   Quantity

And another formula that may be used is:

$$\frac{\text{Percent Solution on Hand}}{\text{Percent Solution Wanted}} \times \text{Amount of Solution on Hand} = \text{Total Amount of New Solution}$$

To then find the amount of water to add, simply subtract the amount on hand from the new total.

EXAMPLE: How much water must be added to 100 cc of a 5% solution to make a 1% solution?

NOTE: This type problem usually is stated, "How much water must be added," or "How much of a weaker solution (1%) can be made from a given amount (100 cc) of a stronger solution (5%)."

This problem can be solved by using the second formula shown below:

$$\frac{5}{1} \times 100 \text{ cc} = 500 \text{ cc}$$

Answer: Add enough water (400 cc) to the 100 cc of 5% stock solution to make 500 cc, which will be a 1% solution.

NOTE: Your answer will always be a larger quantity than stated in your problem.

EXAMPLE: How can a 1 : 8000 solution be made from 2 cc of a 1% solution?

In this problem it is probably easier to convert the percentages to fractions and then solve by the formula:

$$\frac{\frac{1}{100}}{\frac{1}{8000}} \times 2 \text{ cc} = \frac{1}{100} \div \frac{1}{8000} \times 2$$

$$= \frac{1}{\cancel{100}} \times \frac{\overset{80}{\cancel{8000}}}{1} \times 2 = 160 \text{ cc}$$

Answer: Add 158 cc water to 2 cc of a 1% solution to make a 1 : 8000 solution.

COMPARISON OF THE TWO SOLUTION FORMULAS

In the problem, "Make a 5% solution of merbromin from 50 cc of a 25% solution," you have a *given amount* of solution from which you are to make a *weaker* solution, so the formula to use would be:

$$\frac{\text{Percent Solution on Hand}}{\text{Percent Solution Wanted}} \times \text{Solution on Hand} = \begin{array}{l} \text{Total Amount of} \\ \text{New Solution} \end{array}$$

or using the proportion formula:

$$\frac{25}{5} \times \cancel{50}^{\,10} \text{ cc} = 250 \text{ cc}$$

Greater : Lesser :: Greater : Lesser
Percent   Percent   Quantity   Quantity

$25\% : 5\% :: x : 500 \text{ cc}$

$5x = 1250$

$x = 250 \text{ cc}$

If this problem had been stated, "Make 1 pint of a 5% solution from a 25% solution," the solution formula shown below would be used:

Drug : Water :: Percent : 100

$x \text{ cc} : 50 \text{ cc} :: 5\% : 25\%$

$25x = 2500$

$x = 100 \text{ cc}$

In this problem you are to make a given amount from an unknown amount.

Answer in First Example: Add 200 cc of water to 50 cc of a 25% stock solution of merbromin to make a 5% solution.

Answer in Second Example: Measure 100 cc of 25% solution of merbromin and add enough water (400 cc) to make a pint of 5% solution.

In the first example, you do not know how much solution you are to make, but you do know how much you have from which to make the unknown total amount. In the second example, you are instructed to make a certain amount, but do not know how much of the stock solution will be needed to make your solution. In other words, in the first example, you are to make an unknown amount of solution from a given amount, while in the second, you are to make a given amount from an unknown amount.

PRACTICE PROBLEMS

1. How much water must be added to a quart of 2% bichloride solution to make a $\frac{1}{2}$% solution?

2. How much of a $\frac{1}{2}$% solution can be made from 200 cc of a 5% solution?

3. Make a 5% solution of merbromin from 100 cc of a 10% solution.

4. How much of a 2% solution can be made from 500 cc of a 1 : 5 solution?

5. How much water must be added to 1 liter of a 10% Lysol solution to make a 1% solution?

6. How much of a 5% solution of sodium chloride can be made from 400 cc of a 25% solution?

7. How much 1 : 1600 solution can be made from 10 cc of a 1 : 16 solution?

8. Make a 3% solution of iodine from 6 oz of a 10% solution.

9. Make a $\frac{1}{4}$% solution of silver nitrate from 1 oz of a 1% solution.

10. Make 1 quart of a 1% solution from a 5% solution.

Answers to Practice Problems

1. Add 3000 cc water to the quart for a total of 1 liter (4000 cc) of $\frac{1}{2}$% solution.
2. 2000 cc. [Add 1800 cc water to the 200 cc of 5% solution.]
3. Add 100 cc water to the 10% solution to make a total of 200 cc of 5% solution.
4. 5000 cc. [Add 4500 cc water to the 500 cc. Note that a 1 : 5 solution = a 20% solution.]
5. Add 9000 cc water to the liter (1000 cc) for a total of 10,000 cc (10 liters).
6. 2000 cc. [Add 1600 cc to the 400 cc of 25% solution.]

7. 1000 cc. [Add 990 cc water to the 10 cc.]
8. 600 cc. [Add 420 cc to the 6 oz (180 cc).]
9. Add 90 cc of water to the 1 oz (30 cc) of 1% solution for a total of 120 cc of $\frac{1}{4}$% solution.
10. 200 cc. [This problem is worked by the other solution formula. It does not say make a 1% solution from a quart of 5% solution. You are to make a quart of a 1% solution; therefore, you will need to determine how much of the 5% solution you will need to make your solution. Answer: Measure 200 cc of the 5% solution, pour into a quart container, and add water to make a quart.]

If you made more than one error, review the lesson and try to solve the problems again.

APPENDIX A

Rules for Giving Medications

1. Read all orders correctly—never guess at what may be intended. Read orders from both cardex and chart. Consult your team leader, head nurse, or instructor if there is any question about an order.
2. Read the order three times to ensure correct interpretation.
3. Read the label three times when preparing medications:
   a. When taking from shelf.
   b. When removing from container.
   c. When returning to the shelf.
4. Think only of what you are doing when pouring medications. Do not talk to anyone, and do not permit anyone to talk to you.
5. Remove the top cap of the bottle and hold between fingers or upside down to prevent getting foreign matter in the bottle.
6. Pour away from label (label should be turned toward palm of hand) to prevent soiling label.
7. Never use a drug from an unmarked bottle.
8. If you mix two medicines and they form a precipitate or change color when mixed, they should not be administered.
9. If there is already a precipitate or sediment in a medication that comes directly from the pharmaceutical company (as in some insulin), roll gently between palms to mix before administering.
10. Measure medications accurately. Use standard graduate measuring glass and hold glass so that line indicating desired dose is at eye level. Do not measure drams with a teaspoon.
11. Never pour medicine back into the bottle.
12. Check patient's identification before giving medicine and remain with patient until medication has been swallowed.
13. Use extreme care in solving all problems. Be sure your answer is correct. Use more than one method to solve problems and have someone else check your answer if you have any doubt about its being correct.

APPENDIX **B**

Summary of the Systems of Measurement

COMPARISON OF METRIC AND APOTHECARIES' SYSTEMS

Metric System

Common units: milligram, gram, cubic centimeter, milliliter, and liter.

Arabic numbers and decimal fractions are used.

The number is *followed* by the abbreviation.

Example: morphine 0.016 g or morphine 16 mg

Apothecaries' system

Common units: grain, minim, dram, and ounce.

Roman numerals and common fractions are used.

Abbreviation or symbol *precedes* the number.

Examples: morphine grain $\frac{1}{4}$, aspirin grain v, ℥ ii (2 drams)

THE METRIC SYSTEM

Dry Weight (Solid) Measure

1000 micrograms (μg) = 1 milligram (mg)

1000 milligrams (mg) = 1 gram (g)

1000 grams (g) = 1 kilogram (kg)

Volume or Liquid Measure

1000 cubic centimeters (cc) or 1000 milliliters (mL) = 1 liter

NOTE: Cubic centimeters and grams are equivalent, since 1 cc weighs approximately 1 g. Cubic centimeters and milliliters are units of liquid measure; grams and milligrams are units of dry (solid) measure. Kilograms are frequently used to determine dosage on the basis of an individual's body weight.

THE APOTHECARIES' SYSTEM

Dry Weight (Solid) Measure	Liquid Measure
60 grains = 1 dram ($\mathfrak{z}$)	60 minims (m) = 1 fluid dram ($f\mathfrak{z}$)
8 drams = 1 ounce (oz or $\mathfrak{z}$)	8 drams = 1 ounce ($f\mathfrak{z}$)
480 grains = 1 ounce	16 ounces = 1 pint (pt or O.)
	2 pints = 1 quart (qt)
	4 quarts = 1 gallon (gal or C.)
	480 minims = 1 ounce

NOTE: *Minims and grains are equivalent, since 1 minim weighs approximately 1 grain. Minim is a unit of liquid measure, and grain is a unit of dry measure.*

HOUSEHOLD MEASURES

60 drops (guttae) = 1 teaspoonful (t or tsp)
4 teaspoonsful = 1 tablespoonful (T or Tbs)
2 tablespoonsful = 1 ounce (oz)
6 ounces = 1 teacupful
8 ounces = 1 glassful or 1 tumblerful
8 teaspoonsful = 1 ounce

EQUIVALENT QUANTITIES AMONG THE THREE SYSTEMS

Household Measures	Apothecaries' System	Metric System
1 teaspoonful	1 dram or 60 minims	4 or 5 cubic centimeters
1 tablespoonful	3 or 4 drams	15 or 16 cubic centimeters
2 tablespoonsful	8 drams or 1 ounce	30 or 32 cubic centimeters
1 teacupful	6 ounces	180 cubic centimeters
1 glassful or 1 tumblerful	8 ounces	240 cubic centimeters

Weight Equivalents

1 gram (g) = 0.035 ounce (oz)
454 grams = 1 pound (lb)
1 kilogram (kg) = 1000 grams = 2.2 pounds

Length Equivalents

1 millimeter (mm) = 0.3937 inch
1 centimeter (cm) = 10 millimeters = 0.3937 inch
25.4 millimeters = 1 inch
2.54 centimeters = 1 inch
1 meter (m) = 100 centimeters = 39.37 inches
1 kilometer (km) = 1000 meters = 0.6214 mile
1.609 kilometer = 1 mile

APPROXIMATE METRIC AND APOTHECARIES' EQUIVALENTS

Metric System	Apothecaries' System

1 milligram (mg) = $\frac{1}{60}$ grain
60 or 64 milligrams* or 0.06 gram = 1 grain
1 gram or milliliter or cubic centimeter = 15 or 16 grains or minims (m)
4 or 5 grams, milliliters, or cubic centimeters = 1 dram or 60 or 64 grains or minims
30 or 32 grams, milliliters, or cubic centimeters = 1 ounce or 8 drams or 480 minims
500 grams, milliliters, or cubic centimeters = 1 pint or 16 ounces
1 kilogram or 1 liter or 1000 milliliters or cubic centimeters = 1 quart
4 liters or 4000 milliliters or cubic centimeters = 1 gallon

NOTE: There are actually 64 mg in 1 grain and 16 grains in 1 g, but, for ease of calculation, the values of 60 and 15 may be used.

---

*The U.S. Pharmacopeia also gives 65 and 66 mg = 1 grain.

The following commonly used equivalents should be memorized:

$$1 \text{ gram} = 1 \text{ milliliter} = 1 \text{ cubic centimeter}$$
$$60 \text{ or } 64 \text{ milligrams} = 1 \text{ grain}$$
$$1000 \text{ milligrams} = 1 \text{ gram} = 15 \text{ or } 16 \text{ grains}$$
$$1 \text{ kilogram} = 2.2 \text{ pounds}$$
$$1 \text{ minim} = 1 \text{ grain}$$

RULES FOR CONVERTING UNITS

Conversion Wanted	Method
Grams to grains or milliliters (or cc) to minims	Multiply by 15 or 16
Grains to grams or minims to milliliters (or cc)	Divide by 15 or 16
Grains to milligrams	Multiply by 60 or 64
Milligrams to grains	Divide by 60 or 64
Milligrams to grams	Move decimal point three places to the *left* (ie, divide by 1000)
Grams to milligrams	Move decimal point three places to the *right* (ie, multiply by 1000)

APPENDIX C

Formulas

1. To determine the number of tablets or capsules:

$$\frac{\text{Amount Ordered}}{\text{Amount on Hand}} = \text{Number Tabs or Caps to Give}$$

2. Dosage formulas:

   a. Drug on Hand : Dilution :: Dose Ordered : x

   b. $\dfrac{\text{Drug Ordered}}{\text{Drug on Hand}} \times \text{Dilution} = \text{Amount to Give}$

3. Insulin dosage formula:

   a. $\dfrac{\text{Units Insulin Ordered}}{\text{Insulin on Hand}} \times 16 \text{ minims} = \text{Number Minims to Give}$

   b. $\dfrac{\text{Dose Ordered}}{5} = \text{Number Units U-500 Insulin to Draw up in a U-100 Syringe}$

4. Preparing antibiotics or drugs in powder form:

   a. $\dfrac{\text{Drug on Hand (Total Amount)}}{\text{Dose Ordered}} \times 1 \text{ mL} = \text{Amount Diluent to Add to Vial of Powder}$

   b. Drug on Hand : x mL :: Amount to be Given : 1 mL
      (Total Amount)

5. Children's dosage:

a. Clark's rule:

$$\frac{\text{Weight of Child}}{150} \times \text{Adult Dose} = \begin{array}{l}\text{Approximate Child's Dose}\\\text{When Weight Is Given}\end{array}$$

b. BSA formula:

$$\frac{\text{Body Surface Area of Child (m}^2) \times \text{Adult Dose}}{1.73} = \begin{array}{l}\text{Approximate}\\\text{Child's Dose}\end{array}$$

c. mg/kg body weight formula:

mg Medication Ordered $\times$ kg Body Weight of Child = Dose for Child

d. Fried's rule:

$$\frac{\text{Child's Age in Months}}{150} \times \text{Adult Dose} = \begin{array}{l}\text{Approximate Dose for}\\\text{Children Under 2 years}\end{array}$$

e. Young's rule:

$$\frac{\text{Child's Age}}{\text{Child's Age} + 12} \times \text{Adult Dose} = \begin{array}{l}\text{Approximate Dose for}\\\text{Children Over 2 Years}\end{array}$$

6. Formulas for administration of IV fluids:

a. To determine total time to be infused:

$$\frac{\begin{array}{c}\text{Total Drops to Be Infused}\\\text{(total mL} \times \text{drop factor)}\end{array}}{\text{Flow Rate (drops/min)} \times 60} = \begin{array}{l}\text{Total Time (in min)}\\\text{Infusion Is to flow}\end{array}$$

b. To determine flow rate in milliliters per minute:

$$\frac{\text{Total Milliliters Ordered}}{\text{Total Minutes to Flow}} = \text{Milliliters per Minute}$$

c. To determine flow rate:

$$\text{Flow Rate (drops/min)} = \frac{\begin{array}{c}\text{Total Volume} \times \text{Drop Factor}\\\text{(drops/mL)}\end{array}}{\text{Total Infusion Time (min)}}$$

$$\text{Flow Rate (mL/min)} = \frac{\text{Drops per Minute}}{\text{Drop Factor}}$$

d. Flow rate for infants:

$$\text{Flow Rate (microdrops/min)} = \frac{\text{Total Volume} \times \text{Drop Factor (microdrops/mL)}}{\text{Total Infusion Time (min)}}$$

7. Formulas for calculating IV medications:

a. $\dfrac{\text{Total Volume (mL)}}{\text{Total Infusion Time}} \times \text{Drop Factor} = \text{Flow Rate (or drops/min)}$

b. $\dfrac{\text{Total Volume (mL)}}{\text{Total Amount Medication}} \times \text{Drop Factor} \times \text{Dose Ordered/min} = \text{Flow Rate}$

c. Total Amount Medication : Total Solution :: Dose Ordered : x
(Answer will be in mL; multiply by drop factor to obtain flow rate.)

d. $\dfrac{\text{Total Medication Prescribed}}{\text{Prescribed Time for Administration}} = \text{Amount Received per Minute}$

8. Formulas for preparation of solutions:

a. To solve for amount of drug, amount of water, and percentage strength using pure (100%) drugs:

Drug : Water :: Percent : 100

or,

$$\frac{\text{Desired Strength}}{\text{Available Strength}} = \frac{\text{Amount to Use}}{\text{Amount to Make}}$$

b. To make a given quantity of a weaker solution from a stronger solution when two percents, two ratios, or a ratio and percent are given:

Drug : Water :: % Solution Wanted : % Solution on Hand

c. To make a weaker solution from a *given* amount of a stronger solution:

Greater % : Lesser % :: Greater Quantity : Lesser Quantity

9. To change Celsius to Fahrenheit:

$$(°C \times \frac{9}{5}) + 32 = °F$$

To change Fahrenheit to Celsius:

$$(°F - 32) \times \frac{5}{9} = °C$$

APPENDIX D

Abbreviations and Symbols Used in the Text

Abbreviation	Latin Derivation	Meaning
ac	*ante cibum*	before meals
bid	*Bis in die*	twice a day
BSA		body surface area
c̄		with
cap		capsule
cc		cubic centimeter
D/S		dextrose in saline
D/W		dextrose in water
elix		elixir
g		gram
grain		grain
guttae	*guttae*	drop
(H)		by hypodermic
hs	*hora somni*	at bedtime
IM		intramuscularly
IV		intravenously
kg		kilogram
lb		pound
m		minim
m^2		square meter
mEq		milliequivalent
mg		milligrams
min		minute
mL		milliliter
oz		ounce

NPH		isophane insulin
pc	*post cibum*	after meals
po	*per os*	by mouth
prn	*pro re nata*	when necessary
PZI		protamine zinc insulin
qd	*quaque die*	every day
q hr	*quaque hora*	every hour
qid	*quator in die*	four times a day
s̄		without
sol		solution
sc		subcutaneously
ss	*semis*	one-half
stat	*statim*	at once
t		teaspoon
T		tablespoon
tab		tablet
tid	*ter in die*	three times a day
U		unit
USP		United States Pharmacopeia

Symbols Used

ʒ = dram

℥ = ounce